Endomorph Plan For Women

A Step-by-Step Guide for your Specific Body Type to Weight Loss with Delicious Recipes and Specified Exercises

Lucy J. Bell

Lucy J. Bell

Endomorph Diet Plan For Women

© Copyright 2020 by Lucy J. Bell
All rights reserved

This document is geared towards providing exact and reliable information with regards to the topic and issue covered. The publication is sold with the idea that the publisher is not required to render accounting, officially permitted, or otherwise, qualified services. If advice is necessary, legal or professional, a practiced individual in the profession should be ordered.

From a Declaration of Principles which was accepted and approved equally by a Committee of the American Bar Association and a Committee of Publishers and Associations.

In no way is it legal to reproduce, duplicate, or transmit any part of this document in either electronic means or in printed format. Recording of this publication is strictly prohibited and any storage of this document is not allowed unless with written permission from the publisher. All rights reserved.

The information provided herein is stated to be truthful and consistent, in that any liability, in terms of inattention or otherwise, by any usage or abuse of any policies, processes, or directions contained within is the solitary and utter responsibility of the recipient reader. Under no circumstances will any legal responsibility or blame be held against the publisher for any reparation, damages, or monetary loss due to the information herein, either directly or indirectly.

Respective authors own all copyrights not held by the publisher.

The information herein is offered for informational purposes solely, and is universal as so. The presentation of the information is without contract or any type of guarantee assurance.

The trademarks that are used are without any consent, and the publication of the trademark is without permission or backing by the trademark owner. All trademarks and brands within this book are for clarification purposes only and are owned by the owners themselves, not affiliated with this document.

Lucy J. Bell

Disclaimer

All erudition contained in this book is given for informational and educational purposes only. The author is not in any way accountable for any results or outcomes that emanate from using this material. Constructive attempts have been made to provide information that is both accurate and effective, but the author is not bound for the accuracy or use/misuse of this information. Therefore, before deciding to undertake any nutritional path, it would be better to consult your doctor of trust.

Table of contents

Introduction 6
Endomorph Diet 8
How To Follow The Endomorph Diet 24
Meal Planning 42
   A 7-day Sample Menu 48
Simple Exercise For Your Body Type 93
Healthy Eating Habits 117
Endomorph Recipes 134
How To Speed Up Metabolism 182
Conclusion 211

Introduction

Endomorphs are people who work hard but fail to lose body fat. An endomorph is someone who has a sluggish metabolism and is genetically inclined to store fat easily. Endomorphs are typically wide framed with medium to large joints, but not always. Endomorphs also have varying degrees of sensitivity to carbohydrates and insulin resistance, so high carbohydrate diets are typically not successful for regulating body fat. Processed and unprocessed carbohydrates containing white sugar and white flour are particularly harmful to endomorphs and appear to convert to body fat more quickly. Low to moderate diets with high protein carbohydrates typically perform well for endomorphs.

Although some genetically gifted mesomorphs and ectomorphs can eat whatever they want and never gain any weight, the endomorph has to eat something clean and healthy almost all the time. That requires the creation of high nutritional discipline levels. Endomorphs are the forms that appear to accumulate body fat very easily if they consume too much or if they eat the wrong foods. Endomorphs also cannot "cheat" and get away with it. Their metabolism is incredibly unforgiving.

One or two cheat meals a week are a limit. They are often set back by bad everyday eating habits or regular cheat days.

Endomorphs typically have a very hard time losing weight by dieting alone. Often even an almost ideal diet won't function by itself since endomorphs require the metabolism boost that exercise offers. More essential for the endomorphs is a systematic approach to training and diet regarding fat loss. Even though they have a very difficult metabolism to lose fat, this book contains several exercises and training routines to help them begin to lose weight in at least one week. Following the diet will help you easily lose weight and build the ideal body you so crave.

CHAPTER ONE

Endomorph Diet

An endomorph is one of three body types (somatotypes) identified by an American psychologist William Sheldon in the 1940s. Sheldon theorized the correlation of a person's body type with a form of personality. However, in some circles, the notion of three distinct forms of the human body endures is not generally recognized today. A mesomorph is the "ideal" type of body — strong and muscular, with an average frame and more muscle than fat. Through workout, mesomorphs can quickly put muscle on, but if they don't watch what they eat, they can also add body fat. An ectomorph has a leaner, less natural muscle build than a mesomorph and a lower propensity to weight. Ectomorphs can find it difficult to put on fat or muscle, no matter how hard they work. An endomorph has a higher proportion of body fat than a mesomorph and less muscle mass. Endomorphs tend to have a plumper body shape and are more susceptible to calorie use. They can quickly gain weight, prefer to accumulate fat and will have a tougher time losing weight.

People with a form of endomorphic body appear to have a sluggish metabolism, making it easier for them to gain weight and more difficult for them to lose. This stunts muscle development as well. However, people with endomorphic bodies will also achieve and sustain their health goals by adopting a particular diet and exercise schedule. People with endomorphic bodies typically have smooth, round bodies with a small waist and large bones, joints, and hips irrespective of their height. This book deals with what an endomorphic diet is, including what to consume and avoid. This book also talks about workouts that can help people with endomorphic bodies lose weight and build muscle.

Ever wondered why some people could eat absolutely anything and never put on weight, while others can get overweight just from the scent of chocolates and cookies? Well, the response to that lies in each individual's body form. The three body forms are Ectomorph, Endomorph, and Mesomorph, and these are primarily responsible for the pattern your body stores and burns fat. Read on to learn more about your body type.

Get to Know Your Type

Some personal coaches and bodybuilding centers use a general description of your body type to determine your needs and personal objectives. Your body type depends on your bone structure and body frame. Hence, each form responds to exercise and diet differently. You need to know your body type to get the full benefits of your workout routine and diet.

The Skinny Ones - Ectomorph

Do you feel like a skinny bone bag and your chest is just as flat as the floor on which you walk? If YES, then you are among the category of Ectomorph Body.

The Ectomorphs with small bones, slender joints and muscles, are slim, strong and short. They have a delicate, soft, and linear physique. Ectomorphs are not naturally strong, and they have to work hard to build muscles and gain strength. They have a superfast metabolism. They can eat all day while never adding weight.

Simple Ectomorphic Features

Slight build, flat chest, lean body, lightly muscled, slim and slender. An individual with these features takes more time in building muscles and does not easily gain weight.

Ectomorphs should focus on building lean muscle mass by weight lifting and aerobic exercises (this applies to women). Since Ectomorphs have little strength, they can only do mild exercises and rest between sets. Running on the treadmill, running, weight lifting exercises, crunches, and cycling are the perfect activities for people with these body styles.

If they want to gain some weight and develop muscle, ectomorphs can eat about 3000 and 3500 calories a day. They can consume 5-6 meals a day and include more carbohydrates and protein-rich foods in their diet, such as green vegetables, whole grain bread, legumes, dairy products, chicken and red meats.

The Endomorph - Short & Curvy

Unlike Ectomorphs, it is difficult for Endomorphs to lose weight, and they are often overweight. They have a round face, large bones, large hips and thighs. Owing to a slower metabolism, endomorphs find it difficult to burn calories and usually have a high degree of fat around their midsection.

Do not be disappointed if this describes you, as Endomorphic body types have their advantages; Endomorphs are naturally muscular and receive full value from muscle-building programs.

Simple Endomorphic Features

Bulky and round body, can easily put on weight, especially around the middle area. Generally short, slow metabolism, build muscle fast, often overweight and obese.

To control your metabolism, you should eat small meals regularly. Take a good diet and never starve yourself to weight loss. People with this type of body can reduce their carbohydrate intake and eat more protein-rich foods. Proteins help keep your muscles healthy and keep you satiated for longer hours.

Endomorphs benefit from aerobic exercise and weight training and can thus easily build muscle. For Endomorphs, the ideal workout regimen will involve aerobic workouts and weight training. Other workouts, like Pilates, Yoga, and Aerobics, can be of great benefit as well.

The Mesomorph - Sporty Body

These are the people who are blessed with the best form of body — well-defined muscles, big bones and a great physique. You'll have a well-developed chest, wide shoulders, a slimmer waistline, strong belly and toned thighs if you're a Mesomorph.

What else would one ask for? However, there is a downside: Mesomorphs have limited versatility and need to engage further in versatility preparation.

Mesomorphic Core Features

Strong build, full of energy, and willing to do a lot of physical activity. Females have an hour-glass figure while males have a rectangular form, muscular and toned body, excellent physical fitness and easy muscle gain with proper training.

Mesomorphs should eat a protein-rich diet and slow-absorbing carbohydrates, including vegetables, brown rice, fish, eggs, legumes and olive oil. Ideally, their fitness schedule should be a mix of interval training, high-intensity aerobic training, moderate weight training, core training and strength training.

What is an Endomorphic Diet?

Endomorphic diets and fitness strategies have been created by experts to work with and against to help people with endomorphic bodies lose weight or maintain healthy body weight. People with endomorphic bodies appear to have a slower metabolism, likely because of their more substantial structure. A slower metabolism can result in the body becoming more likely to turn excess calories into fat. Thus, people with endomorphic bodies can monitor what they eat, what they eat, and how much they eat.

Individuals with endomorphic bodies, according to Sheldon, can also have characteristics that make pursuing diets and exercise plans more difficult. They may, for example, have a general desire for food, warmth and relaxation. These people often typically have a larger build and bear more weight to be more sedentary. It can be difficult for them to gain muscle mass since excess body fat causes hormone estrogen release. Increases in estrogen levels tend to decrease hormone levels, which promote muscle development, such as testosterone.

What Does an Endomorph Eat While Losing Weight?

If you have an endomorphic body, losing weight can be more challenging to you than someone with a mesomorphic body. But it doesn't mean that you can't do it. No matter what sort of body you have, there is only one way of losing weight: losing more calories than eating. As long as you do this, you'll lose weight no matter what kinds of food you consume.

Variation in Endomorph Guidelines

One proposed endomorphic diet emphasizes lean protein, healthy fats and complex carbs (as in diets in the Mediterranean, paleo, and keto) and restricts simple carbs such as white bread, added sugars, and processed food. Overall, this advice is beneficial for everyone, not just endomorphs.

It is beneficial because healthy fats, such as olive oils, avocados, and fatty fish such as salmon, are satiating, while complex carbs such as whole grains and veggies are slow-burning energy sources. Simple carbs such as candy and starchy foods are easy to burn, promoting a higher intake of calories, and contributing to weight gain.

In general, people with endomorphic bodies will benefit from a diet plan that includes healthy fats, proteins, and carbohydrates from fruits, vegetables, and high-fiber, unrefined foods. Some examples of protein-rich foods or balanced monounsaturated and polyunsaturated fats include:

- ❖ Low-fat dairy products, including low-fat milk, yogurt, and cheeses
- ❖ Meats, such as chicken and turkey
- ❖ Most types of fish, fatty fish in particular
- ❖ Most non-tropical vegetable oils, especially olive, canola and avocado oil
- ❖ Most non-tropical vegetable oils, especially olive, canola and avocado oil
- ❖ Egg whites and white eggs
- ❖ Most nuts, including almonds, hazelnuts, and walnuts

Some examples of carbohydrates suitable for endomorphic diets include:

- ❖ Dried beans and legumes, such as lentils, kidney beans and chickpeas

- ❖ Fruits, like pineapple and melons
- ❖ Non-starchy vegetables like broccoli and celery
- ❖ Full-grain or whole-grain goods, such as all-grain cereal and 100% stone-ground whole-grain bread
- ❖ Some starchy vegetables, including sweet potatoes, yams, maize and carrots
- ❖ Some starchy, unrefined vegetables such as quinoa and amaranth

People with an endomorphic body type appear to be more susceptible to carbohydrates and insulin, according to the American Council on Exercise (ACE). Insulins are hormones that help the cells to reach blood sugars.

Thus, people following an endomorphic diet may want to restrict or avoid dense carbohydrate foods, specifically refined carbohydrates, sugar and white flour. Carbohydrate-rich foods release carbohydrates easily into the bloodstream, causing spikes and dips in blood sugar. The body is also more likely to transform these sugars into fat than to use them as energy.

Endomorphic bodies often have a higher risk of turning excess calories into fat. For the same cause, people adopting an endomorphic diet may also want to avoid foods rich in calories but weak in nutrients.

Some examples of foods on the endomorph diet to limit or avoid include:

- ❖ White bread, white rice, fresh bagels, and pasta
- ❖ Spaghetti, chocolate and other treats
- ❖ Products and boiled cakes
- ❖ Soft drinks, sports drinks, energy drinks
- ❖ Processed cereals, such as bran flakes, instant oatmeal and puffed rice
- ❖ Highly refined and fried food
- ❖ Rich milk products, including yogurt, whipped cream and ice cream
- ❖ Red Flesh
- ❖ Sodium-rich foodstuffs
- ❖ Alcoholics
- ❖ Fried saturated fat oils, such as palm or coconut oil

What Activities do Endomorphs do Best?

Every good weight loss plan should involve physical exercise such as cardio training and strength training, irrespective of the body type. One type of exercise that could be considered by an endomorph (or someone else) is HIIT, which stands for high-intensity interval training. Instead of only jumping on a treadmill and jogging for as long as possible (also known as low-intensity steady-state exercise, or LISS), HIIT includes raising the heart rate with vigorous activity like sprinting, interspersed with lower-intensity jogging or walking rest times. You can sprint for a minute in a typical HIIT session and slow down to a jog or walk for another minute, before sprinting again, for a maximum of 20 minutes overall.

Equally relevant for weight loss is strength training, such as weightlifting. Lean muscle burns body fat, so the leaner muscle you've got, the more effective you'll be at weight loss. But it is important to speak with your healthcare provider before beginning any new diet plan or workout regimen, no matter what your body type or fitness goal is. Exercise is an important part of any weight-loss strategy, especially for people with a form of an endomorphic body. Exercising helps to improve metabolism and decrease fat.

Cardiovascular activities, like running, can burn calories and lead to a calorie deficit. It means that everyone uses more calories than they eat, and probably burns excess fat. The ACE suggests that people with an endomorphic body should adopt "fully balanced" workout routines concentrating on cardiovascular and strength training.

Examples of good cardiovascular workouts include:

- ❖ High-intensity interval training (HIIT): a person may alternate in HIIT between periods of very high-intensity exercise and low-intensity exercise or rest time. Those with endomorphic bodies should try to do HIIT sessions for 30 minutes per day, two or three times a week.

❖ Stable State Training (SST): Longer sessions of regular exercise of moderate to low intensity; good activities on SST include walking, jogging, and swimming. People with a form of endomorphic body can try to do SST sessions of 30–60 minutes two to three times a week.

Strength and weight exercises are an important part of virtually every weight loss strategy, particularly for endomorphic body type people. These people also have a low percentage of muscle mass, but they usually have large, thick bones capable of supporting large, heavy muscles. They also appear to have excess body fat, which causes the body to release estrogen, decrease testosterone levels, and impede muscle development. However, healthy muscle tends to improve metabolism, since unlike fat cells, even while resting, muscle tissues consume calories. They allow the body to use fat as fuel, too. Various weight lifting routines and exercises support people with endomorphic bodies. Experts prefer to prescribe activities containing chemicals, for example. Compound exercises together utilize various body tissues and components, which promote control of the body. Most of these exercises can be performed from a standing position using free weights, bodyweight, or barbells.

Some examples of exercises involving compounds include:

Hip hinge or deadlift

To do this:

1. Stand apart with the legs hip-width, above the barbell.
2. Drive the hips back while bracing the neck, retain gentle tension in the back and knees, and lower the floor's heels.
3. Try shooting the hips into the floor, as the bar hits the knees.
4. Finish up tall while the gluts clench.

Pushups

To do this:

1. Place your hands on the floor, spreading your fingers loosely, directly beneath your shoulders.
2. Pack the shoulders while squeezing the gluts and pressing the heels away.
3. Holding the head in line with the body, bend the elbows and guide down the chest toward the floor.
4. Keep the back straight, then strike the hips, gluts, and shoulders to push the chest up.

Squatting

To do this:

1. Stand apart with the legs shoulder-width, push the feet into the floor and turn the hips on.

2. Little by little, and with precision, lower the tailbone with an erect and engaged torso towards the floor.
3. When lowered, slowly push the body away from the floor until the torso is fully extended to stand tall.

<u>Circuit training</u>

Another category of strength exercise that experts recommend is circuit training for people with an endomorphic body type. Circuit training involves doing short, intense workout bouts with tiny rest periods in between.

One example of circuit training could include:

1. Overhead press squat (50 seconds)
2. Rest (10 Sec)
3. Stationary lunge with lateral lift, front right leg (50 seconds)
4. Rest (10 Sec)
5. Stationary lunge with lateral lift, left front leg carrying dumbbells (50 seconds)
6. Rest (10 Sec)
7. Plié squat, dumbbells, or kettlebell (50 seconds)
8. Rest (10 Sec)
9. Push-ups with knee drives on one leg (50 seconds
10. Rest (10 Sec)
11. Triceps plank extension, dumbbells (50 seconds)
12. Rest (10 Sec)
13. Alternate hammer curling step-ups, dumbbells (50 seconds)

14. Repeat these steps thrice

If you have a tough time losing fat and getting lean even though you have a muscular build, you most definitely fall into the endomorph body type category. There are three main categories of the body people fall into:

- ❖ Ectomorphs, slender with a small amount of fat and not much muscle
- ❖ Mesomorphs, muscular and flexible-athletic type
- ❖ Endomorphs, more fat than muscles

Each form of the body must be handled very differently.

You may have been overweight all your life if you're an endomorph, and couldn't imagine being fit and slim. Some endomorphs remain slim and healthy until they reach middle age. Women falling into this type of body would also go through dramatic changes after having their first child. Priorities alter, and as they become less active, their metabolism slows.

Endomorphs appear to have lower bodies, which are solid. While having deltoids (shoulder muscles) built under them, their arms are well built. Their head, hands, upper arms, knees, hips and stomach bear their fat. They have some pretty good calves and thigh muscles. The most beneficial fitness plans should resolve their limitations, and at the same time, improve their strengths.

Endomorphs must adhere to a strict diet regimen intended to minimize their body fat. Unfortunately, since they have a sluggish metabolism, their fat reserves are hard to empty. They'd burn muscle rather than fat. They can never go on a diet without having incorporated an exercise schedule.

The good news is endomorphs quickly develop muscle. Stick with the compound exercises to remove fat during muscle building. The only exercise you can do in isolation is for the deltoids. Trim as much fat off your body before getting into the more advanced workouts.

A workout example will be:

- Monday - Complex exercises in the upper body
- Tuesday - Cardio (not more than 30 minutes)
- Wednesday - Day off
- Thursday - Lower body exercises combination
- Friday - Cardio (30 minutes or less)
- Saturday/Sunday - Day off

With the aid of reducing 500 to 1,000 calories in your daily diet, this exercise will drastically reduce your fat stores. Eat six small meals a day before going to bed and refrain from eating for three hours. If you're an endomorphic body type, give this one a shot.

CHAPTER TWO

How To Follow The Endomorph Diet

Ectomorphs were the leanest and of the least shape in Sheldon's system, with long limbs. Often felt they were more likely to be introverted, imaginative and nervous. Mesomorphs retain builds of the moderately muscular body that were not as lean as the bodies of ectomorphs. Often, they were conceived as being more likely to be bold and assertive. Sheldon described endomorphs with wider hips and jolly, warm personalities as being the roundest. Ectomorphs would be seen as underweight by today's standards, mesomorphs would be slightly underweight, and endomorphs would be very common.

According to the endomorphic diet, people with a higher proportion of body fat or a rounder physique have slower metabolisms, so they are more likely to turn the so-called "excess calories" into fat. The weight loss recommendation for endomorphs is to change their food intake to counteract their bodies' inclination to harbor extra weight. This classification scheme has many issues, and every diet is intended to fix body type or shape.

Body Type Does Not Equal Function

First, saying how people look is a representative of how their bodies function is risky because it is impossible to look at anyone and determine their well-being. People's body sizes are dictated not only by their metabolisms but also by several factors, such as the drugs they take and the amount of physical activity they engage in. It's wrong to recommend a nutritional plan for anyone dependent on their body appearance.

We cannot change our body shape

A second troublesome concept of the endomorphic diet is that the human body's form can be modified. While our physical size and shape are influenced by diet and exercise, it is likely that only within those criteria would. For example, we won't get shorter or taller, we won't develop bigger breasts, and without surgical intervention, we're unlikely to change our bodies' general shape. Thinking that our bodies are inherently malleable and that fulfilling a culturally prescribed standard of beauty would not only offer us greater health but also pleasure. Endorse what body image experts call the illusion of transformation, that body shape or style can be transformed, or that our lives will be changed unambiguously for the better.

What we consume is not about our weight

The endomorphic diet often believes a clear relationship exists between what we eat and our weight and form. Mainstream sources recommend endomorphs gain from a diet plan containing healthy fats, proteins, carbohydrates from fruits, vegetables, and high-fiber, non-refined foods. White bread, highly processed foods, soda and sports drinks, and oils rich in saturated fats are among the food being advised to avoid.

There is nothing objectionable about these guidelines, apart from the fact that they do not necessarily relate more to one form of the body than another. And there's no reason to think they can change your body shape substantially in any discernible manner.

What you weigh is not your fault

Perhaps the most troubling possible effect of diets such as the endomorphic diet is perpetuating the cultural misconception that if they maintain a comparatively higher weight, it is the individual's fault. It over-simplifies nuanced psychological and physiological phenomena and provides false grounds for weight stigma and prejudice toward people perceived to be overweight. (These are prejudices that are not covered in 48 US states by regulation or legislation).

Furthermore, like many food patterns, the endomorphic diet provides the illusion of a cure to an issue many people believe they have, namely their body shape. However, clinical trials testing these claims and published studies investigating this diet's effects for individuals with a specific body shape are absent. Somatotype may represent certain physical health processes, but much further study is required before suggesting specific dietary changes for particular body types would make sense.

Part of me wants the endomorphic diet (or any diet) to be as easy and successful as it is always conceived to be. If Summer could consume less white bread and more vegetables to resolve her self-conscious feelings about her body, I would suggest that she do it. But we all know there is no empirical evidence to indicate this is how our bodies work. I think Summer also knows she and her dress were stunning, and on her wedding day, she glistened with happiness. No diet is the product of that kind of radiance.

Endomorph Diet for Women

The Endomorph diet is ideal for women of any age because of the many benefits of the foods abundant in antioxidants, vitamins, minerals, good fats (omega-3, CLA etc.), complex carbohydrates, animal and plant protein, etc.

Endomorph diet is neither vegan nor vegetarian. Compared with other 'meat' and related diets, beef is not consumed much, but other types of protein-rich food are consumed in almost every meal:

- ❖ Eggs in organic form (omega 3)
- ❖ Cottage cheese and low fat
- ❖ Greek milk and pasta
- ❖ Dairy
- ❖ Fish and Geese
- ❖ Fruits and vegetables

Considerable sources of complex carbohydrates are grains, fruits, and whole grain products. Carbohydrates are consumed in greater amounts than is recommended today in a classic Endomorph diet. It is important to note that carb sources such as whole grain pasta, couscous, potatoes and the likes are not removed, only the quantities are decreased. These types of foods are very small — even omitted — if you have a desk job, endomorphic body form.

Plants as Sources of Protein

Plants are frequently ignored as protein sources (except for vegans, of course), but on Endomorph diet, you can eat at least 30-40 g of protein from plants a day. And this protein will be eaten in 4-7 meals, often combined with animal feed protein. For example, if your target is to eat 2 g of protein per 1 kg of your body weight (1 g per 1 pound of your body weight) and you're 60 kg high, then 40 g of plant protein is around one- third of your expected daily intake of protein. And it is not something that should be ignored. Eating leafy and green vegetables combined with different beans is considered voluminous meals. It provides steady nutrient flow and energy when digested, and keeps you satiated for a long time. If you were dieting and determined to lose some weight (body fats, not just bodyweight), eat foods that are both very voluminous and very low in calories to lose weight.

The need for energy varies with each day. Having a gym workout combined with 1h walking and not doing any physical activity is not the same; thus calories differ from day-to-day. The easiest way to plan your diet is to raise your carbohydrates on heavy physical activity days and decrease them if you are not physically active. A healthy starting point for low-calorie days and low-carbohydrate days is about 50 g of carbs a day. This amount will allow you to easily arrange your diet—all the carbs will come from vegetables and some fruits, while you stay away from ketosis. On days with high carbohydrates, you can eat more carbs during your workouts to have enough energy for scheduled workouts and after workouts to encourage body recovery and regeneration.

Best Diet for Women

What's a woman's best diet? It's like wondering what the right weight loss workout is. There are many solutions, and they may all be equally correct as well as wrong.

We are all different, not just in terms of gender but in terms of age, weight, body shape, body structure, eating and other behaviors, religions, community, aspirations, job/school, etc. So, what's good for you needn't be good for me. Anyway, it is shown that the Endomorph diet, whether cycling carbs or not, promotes optimal health and well-being in several instances. If you're careful about calories, this type of diet will also help you lose fat and lower your overall body weight. Endomorph diet is also advised for women who are trying to conceive, become pregnant, or after pregnancy, trying to get in shape. Why is the Endomorph Diet 'so good'?

- ❖ One absorbs loads of antioxidants, minerals and vitamins
- ❖ A lot of fibers not only support the protection of the digestive system but also reduce LDL cholesterol and increase the cholesterol ratio between LDL and HDL
- ❖ Complex carbs provide constant energy, without burning out

- ❖ Protein helps fix and rebuild the body (to make it easier, of course)
- ❖ Safe fish fats, fish oils, organic eggs, nuts, olive oil, etc. boost the skin, hair, nails, joints, lungs, and various organs

Endomorph diet isn't a Spartan diet, nor do you eat olive oil-soaked fish all day long. It is recommended that you shop cautiously about the foods you consume and their quantities. Here and there, cheat meals will only help you meet your goals and have the Endomorph Diet as a lifestyle. Would you like some wine for dinner? OK, have a glass of wine here and there, but the 'glass of wine here and there' means 0.2 - 0.3l of white or red wine once or twice a week, preferably with some fish, lemon, extra virgin olive oil and plenty of green and leafy vegetables. If you're trying to lose weight, yeah, have that glass of wine, but forget anything that includes carbohydrates other than vegetables. That means you won't be eating whole grain bread, whole grain pasta, potatoes, etc. for that meal.

All should be equilibrated. And if you like wines such as blackberry wine (try to find one from wild blackberries), you'll do much better than drinking those wines often.

Supplements for Women

Unfortunately, we do not continuously have the luxury of eating on time and eating whatever we want. So, feel free to have Meal Replacement Powder (MRP) shakes here and there to keep yourself away from fast foods and similar unhealthy foods. Be vigilant with your macros, and you're going to be doing great. On the other side, whatever supplement companies suggest, MRPs are fine, but they can't fully substitute the right meal, even if you're taking them with greens, multivitamin and multi-mineral capsules, omega-3 pills, Calcium pills, etc. Again, MRPs are fine, but I prefer to eat, for example, a few grilled sardines with spinach and some olive oil and a few drops of lemon instead of powdering with some tablets. With high BV and PDCAAS, whey protein is a great source of fast digestion of protein. It can only be used during workouts and may be combined with foods in different smoothies that will reduce its digestion rate — mix it with bananas, cottage cheese, peanut butter and similar foods.

Just take some nutrients when you need them. For example, joint support supplements facilitate the recovery and regeneration of broken joints and help healthy joints remain healthy. But Endomorph diet includes many of the same Ingredients (among many other benefits), which are also very good for joint health.

Organizing Endomorph Diet

Losing fats (not just losing weight) is a state of mind. You have to change your mind before you change your body, and that cannot happen overnight. If you want to move from A to B, you must follow the strategies used on point B. If you don't alter something (your diet, physical activity, etc.), don't anticipate any improvements, at least not for the better.

As nutrients vary from day to day, they also differ in protein, fats and fibers. Knowing how to gather meals that are perfect for you and your needs is crucial in the daytime. Overall:

- ❖ The bulk of carbs are consumed at breakfast.
- ❖ Carbohydrates are reduced as the day goes by, and fats are increased.
- ❖ Proteins (both from plant and animal protein sources) are consumed in each meal.
- ❖ The meal needs better digestion of fibers, except PWM.
- ❖ Consume at least 4-5 (or more) small meals - this will make the metabolism quicker. It is also much better to get hungry for maybe an hour 4 times a day than twice a day.

- ❖ Eat your fruits as snacks 30-60 minutes before the main meals if you have time. Fruit will make you feel less hungry; it's filled with vitamins, minerals, enzymes, fibers, etc. Only stop fruits containing tons of carbohydrates (if you want to lose weight) or use restraint.
- ❖ Prepare many meals for later use while cooking, and keep them in plastic hermetic pots in the fridge.

These days, everybody is talking about easy weight loss, how to do it, where to go to do it and what are the best ways to rapidly lose weight. Each of us has various reasons why we want to lose those fats, but we're all coming down to one key reason, and that's to alleviate the feeling of having the extra weight turning into something else.

In fast fat loss, most people turn to take food supplement pills marketed on televisions saying you're guaranteed to lose weight within a certain amount of time if you take their pills every day. But if you ask those people if they very quickly got the results, I bet none of them would even answer yes. Why?

Since weight loss doesn't require us to spend money on those supplements, we need to eat and exercise the right way. Another myth about rapid fat loss is that if we buy equipment to help lose those fats or go to the gym every day, we're expected to look fantastic in only a couple of weeks. We also invest time or money on products that promise quick fat loss. If we don't control ourselves and learn how to take care of our bodies, there will still be a fat gain to make us feel less positive.

By adopting a good diet program tailored for our body, we can lose weight more easily than most people who choose to waste time and money on gymnastics, nutritional supplements and other fast fat loss fads. Let's say you are born with a large bone structure like that of an endomorph, no matter how hard you try, you can't be as thin or slim as an ectomorph. You are born with a large bone structure that it doesn't make sense to aspire to appear as slim as an ectomorph. Not only are you wasting your time trying hard to fit in with the form of the body of the ectomorphs, but you are also placing your well-being at risk by adopting diet plans that are not acceptable for you.

Regular exercise is another consideration we should remember when speaking of fast fat loss; sure, it helps to lose weight quickly, but without proper diet, it wouldn't make any real sense either; the fat will still be back to annoy you. So, you're wondering, "What does it take to lose that fat for good?"

The answer is none other than the right diet. Suppose you take good care of your body, then weight loss won't be your problem and never will be your problem. Permanent fat loss only asks you to live healthily; pay attention to what you eat, and you will be in nice shape in no time. If you can do that, you can add the correct dietary workout you are doing for a faster outcome.

Many are actively trying what it takes to lose weight and look lean and sexy. A lot of people wonder how fat from fat cells can be decreased for a thinner appearance. It is essential to remember that weight loss does not mean that you reduce fat in your body.

If you follow a strict diet regime without exercise complementing it, your body will tend to hang on to some amount of fat desperately. Your body tends to change after the initial loss and slow down weight loss quickly. While its percentage can be reduced, it can't be achieved easily in a few weeks. To reach maximum weight loss, you need to increase your physical activity efficiently and change your eating habits. If you're wondering how to minimize fat for a thinner look from the body cells, you need to remember some key physiological factors:

Number of Cells - The amount of fat cells in our body varies widely from person to person. This number is determined by genes and is not subject to alteration. With regular exercise and diet, we can reduce the fat contained in the cells for a slimmer appearance.

Endomorph Body Type - People with the endomorphic body form find it difficult to ease down their percentage. They cannot lose weight as easily as those of other forms of body. By putting a constant demand on the body with the right diet regime and workouts, weight from each body can be reduced. These are some of the efficient ways in which body cells can minimize fat for a thinner look.

Strategies to Accelerate Fat Loss

If you are an endomorph, maybe you have a friend who seems to be able to churn through Big Macs day after day while still retaining a bean pole frame, but with every pound of fat you have lost, you have to scratch and claw. For hard gainers, you don't need yet another post on force-feeding. To mitigate the bad gains and optimize the positive ones (muscle strength), you need an endomorphic diet.

For "fast fat gainers," here are four endomorphic diet strategies:

1. **Cycle Macronutrients**

Completely removing carbohydrates — otherwise known as a bad diet — is painful over time, not just on the brain but on the body. The restrictive diet for too long is certain to fail, and carbs have their place in an athlete's routine. If you're searching for fat loss, you'll need to keep insulin in the bay during the day's inactive hours, which means you're on a carb cycle day (or even days). Insulin is efficient at moving carbs into (healthy) muscle and liver tissue, but it is equally good at pushing carbs into (bad) fat tissue.

Skip the carbohydrates at times farthest from your exercise or sports practices to get the best of both worlds. When sitting all day in the classroom or at work, substitute carbs with healthy fats and keep your protein intake steady. That means something like a three-egg spinach omelet instead of heavy carb-laden pancakes and waffles breakfast. That said, you don't want to completely catabolize the muscle and end up looking like someone fresh off the Survivor cast, by adding carbs before and after your workout to optimize recovery.

2. Fill Up on Veggies

When you're trying to lose weight and also curbing your lion-sized appetite, choosing foods that can satisfy you up without blowing up your calorific needs is important. These foods are an essential component for people who suffer a little more from the deficit determined by the diet. We are discussing foods that have relatively high fiber content and are therefore low in calories. A win-win. That's why staples are non-starchy, high fibrous vegetables such as spinach, kale and broccoli in almost every meal — particularly during a fat loss process.

3. Eat Slowly

You assume, therefore, that you are allergic to carbs (some call it carb intolerant). OK, it might be that you're on to something. Science is beginning to show differences in carb tolerance from one person to another, and everything begins in your mouth. Salivary amylase is an enzyme that begins the digestion of starches in carbohydrates in your saliva. The amylase-forming gene, AMY1, varies in number between individuals. The more you have, the quicker you eat carbohydrates and more efficiently.

Researchers compared 149 Swedish families' genes, which included siblings with a varying body mass index (BMI) of more than 10 kg/m2. AMY1 volume in their saliva was the single biggest factor deciding differences in BMI from one person to the next. What is the solution for those with a reduced presence of this specific gene? Presence during meals, taking time and eating as slowly as possible. Easy in principle, yes, but eating gives your amylase more time to break down the carbs you consume. It evinces the field of play vs. those with more amylase who eat faster.

4. Prioritize Protein

Digesting protein needs a lot more work on the body than fats or carbs. According to CaloriesperHour.com, "nutrition demands the greatest energy expenditure, with figures varying from as high as 30%." It means one can lose up to 30% of the calories you ingest to digest it — plus, protein helps maintain lean body weight. If you're in a calorie deficit, you want to keep as much LBM as you can — not just to look fine, but still perform at your best.

How to Lose Belly Fat

The general census of the United States is growing faster because of processed foods. One of the places where weight is most evident is in the stomach. Men and women both have stomach weight. For men, the last place they normally lose weight is in the stomach. Women have difficulties losing weight in legs and shoulders. Notwithstanding, the reduction of stomach fat requires several essential steps. But in the end, it also means losing weight.

For beginners, dieting is one of the easiest ways to remove stomach weight fat. First, you need to decide how many calories you can eat a day and cut back on it. Cutting your fat intake down is the secret. Today, most foods have names on them. If you make a deliberate effort to halve your fat intake, you will start losing weight. It is possible to produce bigger results by eating less fat. It is best to avoid eating late at night, in addition to reducing calories and fat intake. You need to have at least three hours to eat your last meal or snack before bed. It will be hard to work all the extra calories that you eat at night.

Foods that are rich in carbohydrates should be consumed early in the day rather than at night. Carbohydrates give you the ability to get the day through. You don't need them until you go to bed. Look at the product packets or snacks you consume. Cookies and chips made from potatoes are rich in carbohydrates. If you need a snack at night, find alternatives that are low in fat. Take them out otherwise.

Eighty percent of your beauty is a direct product of your diet. People with endomorphic constructs (naturally heavy people) would have to work harder to remove weight-in-stomach fat. But great strides can still be made by dieting alone. Anyone who wants to get started and lose stomach fat need to start exercising. Don't fall into the trap for all those bogus tummy-reducer goods. By just doing sit-ups or crunches, you won't lose stomach fat. These exercises will help displace fat, but you must still burn off the excess fat through aerobics or cardiovascular exercise.

If necessary, enter a gym. It has a lot of appliances. Start weight lifting and build your muscles to a more athletic physique. Start on the incumbent or stationary bikes to help with fat-burning, particularly if you've never worked out before. Start slowly. It would help if you then started using the treadmill later. You can walk in the evenings if you don't have a gym membership or have no time to enter one. A walk at a good speed through the night will help you burn fat. The classified advertisements for used stationary bikes can also be perused. You do not need to have one that is electronic.

Make diet and exercise a lifestyle. Establish healthy eating patterns. Eat high protein foods and low-fat foods. Eliminate any of the diet bread. Eat foods like rice, chicken, tuna and plenty of vegetables. And cut back on beer that is high in calories.

CHAPTER THREE

Meal Planning

The nutrition you require depends not only on how involved you are and what sport you are playing, but also on your body. Three main forms exist: ectomorph, mesomorph, and endomorph. Below are some diet recommendations for each form, so you can build a meal plan to get and stay in shape for the fuel you need. You may need to make some changes along the way because you may be one sort but have some other characteristics.

Ectomorphs

Typically, ectomorphs are slender individuals with minimal bone structure and limbs. They are usually endurance athletes, with rapid metabolism and high carbohydrate tolerance. They do well when they put in more carbohydrates with normal protein levels and lower fat intake into their diets. The best breakdown: 55% carbohydrates, 25% protein and 20% fat. But don't think about math too much; just concentrate on higher carbohydrates, lower fat. Male ectomorphs must fill their plates with at least three handfuls of carb-related food, two protein palms and two protein palms and two vegetable fists (yes, you must eat your veggies). You may also apply a portion of fat to your thumb. Female athletes should reduce their plate counts by one.

Mesomorphs

Mesomorphs are typically people of medium height with athletic body shapes. They typically have a significant amount of lean mass. Athletes that are mesomorphs are usually active in violent activities, such as wrestling and gymnastics. They prefer to grow muscle and retain a low body fat percentage. A traditional mesomorph diet is more equilibrated than an ectomorph's. Their macro breakdown should be more at 40% sugars, 30% protein and 30% fat. A typical plate will consist of two protein hands, two vegetable paws, two cupped handfuls of carbs, and two fat thumbs for a mesomorph. Again, each portion of female mesomorph athletes should go down by one.

Endomorphs

Endomorphs are typically large-boned and retain both overall body mass and fat mass. A football lineman, or a power lifter, best demonstrates this form. With continuous activity, ectomorphs burn off excess calories, but endomorphs do not burn calories as fast. The calories are stored as fat. You should monitor your carb intake if you're an endomorph, as it can greatly influence your success on the field. Endomorphs typically perform best with higher intakes of fat and protein and closely controlled carb intake (preferably timed with their activity during the day).

The nutritional breakdown should consist of a quantity of proteins 35-40% (kcal), lipids 20-40% (kcal), and, consequently, carb 40-25% (kcal). This is because carbohydrates depend on the amount of lipids, and therefore, when the lipids are at 20%, the carbohydrates will be at 40%, and as the lipids increase, the carbohydrates will drop. A standard plate will consist of two protein hands, two vegetable paws, a cupped handful of carbs and three fat thumbs. Female athletes lower each number down by one. As a society, we have converted dieting into starvation exercise. Rarely do crash diets produce positive results. But a good, planned-out diet meal plan will keep hunger at bay, resulting in gradual and steady weight loss with lasting outcomes. Don't know where to go? Here are a few clues.

Make Protein the Base

Surely a one-size-fits-all diet strategy doesn't work. We have different reactions to food and different age and lifestyle dependent metabolism. But generally speaking, lean protein with any meal still wonders for most people. Load up on protein and fill in gaps from carbohydrates and fats with other macronutrients. Well-balanced diet meal plans contain all three sources but let protein occupy the largest room on your dinner table.

Avoid Fatty Foods

Foods that have so many unhealthy fats like trans and saturated fats are often low in nutrition and high in calories. They're also harmful to your health, increasing your risk of stroke and heart disease. Endomorphs should avoid whole milk products and fried foods and limit their intake of red meat, butter and poultry with the skin to lower saturated fat intake. They should avoid trans fats by avoiding commercial baked goods and any meal containing trans-fats or partly hydrogenated oil. Instead, endomorphs should eat small amounts of healthy fats (lipids) found in plant foods such as avocados, olive oil, walnuts, and fatty fish such as tuna and salmon.

Hungry? Eat Meals With 30/30/8 Grams

Objective: 30 grams of protein per meal, 30 grams of carbohydrates and 8 grams of fat. Consume slow-digesting carbohydrates if it is early in the day. Get your fats from a healthy olive oil teaspoon or a spoonful of good nut butter. This breakdown contains 240 protein and carbs calories (120 calories for both proteins and carbohydrates) and 72 fat calories. Attach some fibrous vegetables to them, and you have a recipe for success.

Eat 4 to 6 times a Day

If you follow the rule 30/30/8 and eat six times a day, the calorie count is slightly below 2000 clocks. Depending on how many calories you consume with exercise, you can find that you need more or less, but this is an excellent starting point. It isn't easy to eat so many times a day, but it's important. Low-calorie meals, like a Denny's Grand Slam breakfast, won't hold you full all day.

Swap out Carbs

This is only if you are a person sensitive to the carb or have no active lifestyle. Hold the protein consumption the same for the last three meals of the day, and double the fat to 16 grams to swap the carbohydrates. To keep you feeling full longer, load up on vegetables. You can still take the carbs during workouts or hard exercise sessions, so keep that in mind when you exercise at night.

Good foods to incorporate

Protein Consumption
- ❖ Skinless chicken breast
- ❖ Extra lean beef
- ❖ Tuna
- ❖ Lean fish (cod, tilapia, halibut, pickerel, etc.)

Carbohydrates
- ❖ Fruit
- ❖ Rice
- ❖ Oatmeal
- ❖ Yam or sweet potato
- ❖ Veggies

Fats
- ❖ Extra virgin coconut oil
- ❖ Macadamia nut oil
- ❖ Extra virgin olive oil
- ❖ Natural butter with peanut, almond or cashew butter
- ❖ Nuts
- ❖ Avocado

A 7-day Sample Menu for the Endomorphic Body Type

DAY 1

Breakfast: *Two scrambled eggs plus one egg white and spinach*

Ingredients

- 1/2 medium onion, separated and sliced into rings
- Two tsp grated parmesan
- 1/2 tsp kosher salt plus a little sprinkle on the onions
- 1/2 tsp black pepper, divided
- One cup fresh spinach leave
- Two medium eggs
- One egg white
- Two tsp olive oil
- 1/2 tsp red pepper flakes

Instructions

- Heat two teaspoons olive oil in a non-stick pan over medium-high heat for about 2 minutes.
- Add the onion slices and sprinkle some kosher salt and a pinch of black pepper. Cook, stirring

- periodically, until golden brown, for about five minutes. Then turn the heat down.
- In a medium cup, whisk the eggs and egg white together, with kosher salt, a pinch of black pepper, and two tsp of Parmesan cheese. Set it aside.
- After the onions are golden brown, add the spinach leaves to the pan. Cook, stirring, for about 1 minute until it begins to wilt.
- Pour the egg mixture into the pan. Cook the eggs over medium heat, guide them back and forth with a rubber spatula until they are set to your taste. Sprinkle with some red pepper flakes. Serve immediately.

Calories: 272Kcal

Snack: *Hummus and Veggies*

Ingredients

- ❖ 1 cup fresh veggies (you can use cucumber, yellow squash, red pepper, baby carrots, and snap peas)
- ❖ 5 ounces precooked chickpeas

- ❖ 1/2 ounce sesame seeds
- ❖ 1/4 cup hot water
- ❖ 1/3 lemon juice
- ❖ 1/3 tbsp Sesame oil
- ❖ 1/2 tbsp Paprika
- ❖ 1/2 garlic clove
- ❖ 1/2 sprig parsley
- ❖ Salt, black pepper to taste

Instructions

- To prepare the hummus, start by peeling the garlic clove, divide it in half to remove the inner core and proceed by chopping it very finely. Then take the sprig of parsley, rinse it, dry it and chop it finely.
- Proceed by preparing the tahini, a typical Middle Eastern sauce (you can also use the one in the market if you prefer). Pour the sesame seeds into a non-stick pan and toast the seeds over low heat for 2-3 minutes. Then transfer them to the mixer to mix the toasted sesame seeds.
- Meanwhile, add the sesame oil, a pinch of salt and the hot water. If you prefer a denser tahini, you can

add more toasted sesame; if more liquid, add more seed oil or hot water.

- Then add the pre-cooked chickpeas, drained from the preservation liquid, and continue to blend. Squeeze the juice of half a lemon and add the garlic, chopped parsley, salt and pepper again.

Once the hummus is ready, you can flavor again with fresh parsley, smoked paprika and a little more seed oil; then your hummus is ready!

Advice:

You can prepare more Hummus at once and refrigerate it for 2-3 days. So, you can use the preparation for many snacks.

Calories: 360kcal

Lunch: *Deli meat wrapped around asparagus spears*

Ingredients

- ❖ 1 tsp olive oil
- ❖ Four asparagus stalks, woody ends trimmed

- ❖ 1/6 package (6 counts) crescent dough
- ❖ 2 ounces deli meat of your choice, sliced thick
- ❖ Salt and pepper to taste
- ❖ 1 tbsp horseradish
- ❖ 2 tbsp shredded Parmesan cheese

Instructions

- Preheat oven to 425°F (214°C) and line the baking sheet with parchment paper.
- In a mixing bowl, add the asparagus to the olive oil and season with salt and Pepper.
- Roll out the crescent dough and force the edges to seal lightly. Split into strips.
- Take the two ounces of deli meat and lay four asparagus spears on top.
- Smear one tbsp horseradish over the length of the asparagus spears and then spread a tbsp of Parmesan cheese.
- Cover the meat tightly around the asparagus spears.
- Moving from top to bottom, wrap the crescent strip around the meat/asparagus bundle in a spiral.
- Place the bundle on a baking sheet, seam side down.

- Bake for 12-15 minutes until the bread is golden brown and the asparagus is tender.

Calories: 369kcal

Snack: *Parmesan chips*

Ingredients

- 1½ oz. parmesan cheese, grated
- 1 tbsp whole flaxseed
- 1/2 tbsp chia seeds
- 1 tbsp pumpkin seeds

Instructions

- Preheat the oven to approximately 180 Celsius degree (350°F).
- Line a baking sheet with parchment paper.
- In a cup, mix the cheese and seeds.
- Pour small piles of mixture onto the pan, leaving some space between them. Do not flatten the piles. Cook for 8-10 minutes. Check frequently the browning of the fries which must be light brown.

- Remove from the oven and wait at least few minutes before serving to let them cool.

Calories: 281kcal

Dinner: *Grilled chicken breast with zucchini noodles and tomato sauce*

Ingredients

- ❖ One large zucchini
- ❖ 5 oz. chicken breast (skinless, boneless)
- ❖ Salt, black pepper

For the Sauce:

- ❖ 1/2 cup chopped tomato (peeled)
- ❖ 1/2 tsp salt
- ❖ Two full tsp oregano
- ❖ 2 tsp minced garlic
- ❖ 2 tsp avocado oil

Instructions

- Preheat the grill pan over medium heat, season the chicken breast with salt and pepper, cook for about 7-8 minutes on each side (if the breast is thin, 5 minutes per side is enough).
- Spiralize your zucchini.
- Preheat the avocado oil in a nonstick pan over medium heat. Add the chopped tomatoes and garlic stir and cook for 3 minutes. Add salt and oregano, stir and cook for 5 minutes.
- Serve the sauce with chicken breasts on top.

Calories: 363kcal

DAY 2

Breakfast: *Cottage cheese with cinnamon and slivered almonds*

Ingredients

- 1/2 cup low fat cottage cheese
- Two tbsp almonds, slivered
- 1/2 cup water

- ❖ Two tbsp oatmeal, raw
- ❖ Cinnamon, to taste

Instructions

- In a bowl, mix oatmeal to 1/2 cup water in a bowl and microwave for about 2 minutes.
- Mix in cottage cheese and microwaved oatmeal and cook again to heat the cottage cheese for 10 seconds.
- Add slivered almonds and sprinkle cinnamon on top

Calories: 305kcal

Snack: *Shelled Sunflower seeds and a variety of pieces of fruits*

Ingredients

- ❖ 4 tbsp strawberries, chopped
- ❖ 1/2 apple (honey crisp or gala), diced
- ❖ 2 tbsp Greek yogurt
- ❖ 1/2 dragon fruit, cubed
- ❖ 3 tbsp roasted, salted sunflower seeds (shelled)

Instructions

- Mix the ingredients (all) in a big bowl. Refrigerate until ready to be served.

Calories: 272Kcal

Lunch: *Fried onion with chicken and peppers on brown rice*

Ingredients

- 1 tbsp vegetable oil, separated
- 2 ounces skinless, boneless chicken breast, cut into strips
- 1/3 cup green onion, chopped
- 4 ounces cooked brown rice
- One clove garlic, minced
- 1/3 red bell pepper, chopped
- 1-ounce frozen peas, thawed
- 1 tsp light soy sauce
- 1 tsp rice vinegar

Instructions

- Heat 1/2 tablespoon veg oil in a skillet on medium heat. Add chicken, clove pepper, green onion, and garlic. Cook and stir till the chicken is cooked through, about five minutes. Remove the chicken from the plate and keep it warm.
- Heat the other 1/2 tablespoon of oil in the same skillet over medium heat. Add rice; cook and stir according to heat. Stir in the soya sauce, the rice vinegar and the peas, and proceed to cook for a minute. Return the chicken mix to the skillet and stir to combine with the rice and heat until ready to serve.

Calories: 336kcal

Snack: *Granola bars with cinnamon berry*

Ingredients

- 1/2 oz. butter, plus extra (greasing)
- 1 tbsp avocado

- ❖ 1/2 cup porridge oats
- ❖ 1 ½ tbsp sunflower seeds
- ❖ 4 tsp sesame seeds
- ❖ 1 ½ tbsp chopped walnuts
- ❖ 2 tsp honey
- ❖ 2 tsp light muscovado sugar
- ❖ 1/2 tsp vanilla extract
- ❖ 1/2 tsp ground cinnamon
- ❖ 1/4 cup dried cranberries, cherries/blueberries, or a mix

Instructions

- Heat oven to 160°C (fan) or 140°C (gas). Butter and line the base of a tin. Mix the seeds, oats, and nuts in the roasting tin, then put in the oven for 5-10 mins to toast.
- Meanwhile, warm the butter, honey, and sugar in a pan, stirring until butter is melted. Add the oat mix, cinnamon, and dried fruit, then mix until all the oats are well coated. Tip into the tin, press down lightly, then bake for 30 mins. Cool in the tin, then cut into four bars.

Advice:

Two bars are the ideal portion for a snack. You can keep the other two bars in the fridge for the next snack.

Calories: 360kcal for a portion (2 bars)

Dinner: *Turkey tacos wrapped in lettuce, diced tomatoes and topped with a slice of avocado*

Ingredients

- One garlic clove, minced
- 3 oz. canned diced tomatoes, drained
- 6 oz. 99% lean ground turkey
- 1 ½ tbsp onion, minced
- 5 oz. butter lettuce (or Romaine)
- 2 tsp taco seasoning
- 1/4 avocado

Instructions

- Heat the skillet over medium-high heat. Add the onion and garlic and brown them. Chop the turkey and cook it on the sauté until it loses its pink color. Add the tomatoes and the taco seasoning.

- Simmer for 4-6 minutes while the sauce thickens. If necessary, add the cornstarch, flour or coconut flour to thicken the sauce.
- Divide the turkey mixture between the lettuce leaves.
- Cut the avocado into pieces and enjoy.

Calories: 314kcal

DAY 3

Breakfast: *Egg frittata made with tomatoes, and baby fresh spinach*

Ingredients

- ❖ Three large eggs, lightly beaten.
- ❖ Two medium tomatoes, diced small
- ❖ 2 cups baby fresh spinach, loosely measured in cup
- ❖ Salt and Pepper, to taste
- ❖ Optionally add extra produce (i.e., zucchini, mushrooms, onions)

Instructions

- In a bowl, beat the three eggs gently with a fork, add salt and pepper to taste, and stir to combine; set aside.
- Heat the stove over medium heat and add the spinach to the pan; leave for about 30 seconds, until slightly wilt.
- Sprinkle the tomatoes and any optional items, add the eggs, cover the pan and cook over medium heat (without stirring) for about 5 minutes or until the edges begin to solidify.
- The omelet is ready. Consume it fresh and soft!

Calories: 268kcal

Snack: *Seed protein bar and apricot*

Ingredients

- 2 tsp hemp protein powder
- 2 tsp oats
- 1 tsp dried cranberries
- 1/4 cup dried apricot

- ❖ 1 tbsp desiccated coconut
- ❖ 1 tsp sesame seeds
- ❖ 1 tsp sunflower seed
- ❖ 1 tsp chia seeds

Instructions

- Blend the dried apricots in a food processor with oats and 30ml boiling water, then transfer in a bowl.
- Toast (over low heat) the sesame seeds, sunflower seeds, and coconut in a non-stick pan. Add the blueberries, apricots, chia seeds, and hemp powder to make a thick paste.
- Leave to cool for 5 minutes but still hot. Take a sheet of cling film on which to spread the mixture, then wrap, close and tighten the sides. Leave in the fridge for about 30 minutes. Then unroll the film and slice to create the bars of the size you prefer.
- The dough, if prepared in larger doses, can be stored in the refrigerator for two weeks.

Calories: 279kcal

Lunch: *Grilled chicken salad with Greek yogurt, tomatoes, and parsley*

Ingredients

- 1 tbsp freshly squeezed lemon juice
- 1 tbsp reduced-fat Greek yogurt
- 1/3 medium cucumber, chopped
- One clove garlic, minced
- Two cherry tomatoes, quartered
- 1/2 medium onion, chopped
- 1/2 tbsp fresh dill, chopped
- 1/2 cup shredded rotisserie chicken
- 1/2 tbsp parsley, chopped
- 1/2 oz feta cheese, crumbled
- Kosher salt, to taste
- Two slices of rye bread

Instructions

- To make the sauce, pour the lemon juice, yogurt, cucumber, and a teaspoon of water into a blender and blend for 30 seconds on high speed. Finish by adding garlic, salt, parsley, and dill. Blend for another 30 seconds. You can add more lemon or water to have less consistency of the sauce to your taste.

- Take a bowl and add the tomato, onion, and feta cheese. Mix and place the two slices of rye on the sides to accompany.
- Pour the sauce over the salad as you like. Enjoy your meal.

Calories: 415kcal

Snack: *Hummus and Veggies*

Follow the procedure already seen on the first day of the meal plan. You can make Hummus directly, only once, with double doses, to use it for two snacks.

Dinner: *Roasted broccoli and cauliflower*

Ingredients

- ❖ 1/2 lb. broccoli, cut into florets
- ❖ 1/2 lb. cauliflower, cut into florets
- ❖ 1/2 lemon (optional)
- ❖ 1 ½ tbsp olive oil or more

❖ Kosher salt to taste

Instructions

- Preheat the oven to 425°F (220°C).
- Arrange the broccoli and cauliflower flowers in a single layer on a baking sheet lined with parchment paper for quick cleaning. Sprinkle with olive oil, then season with kosher salt to taste
- Roast the broccoli and cauliflower for 20 to 25 minutes until crisp with lightly charred edges.
- Squeeze the lemon juice half equally, if desired, and finish with kosher salt to taste. Serve it.

Calories: 291kcal

DAY 4

Breakfast: *Smoothie made with berries, Greek yogurt, and almond milk*

Ingredients

❖ 1/2 cup frozen berries (raspberries, strawberries, blueberries, and/or blackberries)

- ❖ One small banana (optional but adds extra creaminess!)
- ❖ 1/2 cup water or almond milk
- ❖ 5.3 oz. (about 3/4 cup) non-dairy yogurt (prefer plain, but any flavor works fine)
- ❖ 1/2 tsp vanilla extract or granulated vanilla bean powder (optional)

Instructions

- Place the ingredients in a blender, blend until smooth. Stop every now and then and scrape down the sides if necessary. Add an extra splash of milk or water as appropriate.
- If the consistency obtained is more liquid, it can be served in a glass or cup with a straw. If the consistency is more solid, the straw should be replaced by a spoon.

Any way you eat it, top with one or more of these optional toppings (1tbsp):

- ❖ Granola
- ❖ Frozen/fresh berries

- ❖ Cocoa nibs
- ❖ A dollop of your favorite nut butter
- ❖ Chia/hemp seeds
- ❖ Coconut flakes
- ❖ Chopped almonds

Calories: 318kcal (with granola)

Snack: *Lentil hummus and Veggies*

Ingredients

- ❖ 1 cup fresh veggies (you can use cucumber, yellow squash, red pepper, baby carrots, and snap peas)
- ❖ 1/3 cup dried lentils
- ❖ 1/2 tbsp Tahina (If you have it)
- ❖ 1/2 tbsp sweet paprika
- ❖ One wedge lemon juice
- ❖ 1/2 tbsp extra virgin olive oil
- ❖ 1/2 spring parsley
- ❖ 1/2 clove garlic
- ❖ Salt, black pepper to taste

Instructions

To make lentil hummus, check if the lentils you use need to be soaked or not. In case they need soaking, you can soak them in cold water for about 7-8 hours. After the time has elapsed, rinse them very well and pour them into the pot. Cover them abundantly with water. And let them cook for about 45 minutes.

- Once ready, drain and put them inside the blender. Add the clove of garlic, salt, parsley, tahini, paprika, lemon juice, and oil.
- Blend everything for a minute until you get a homogeneous cream. Serve the lentil hummus and add a drizzle of oil and a pinch of paprika.

Advice:

- For a faster version, you can safely use pre-cooked lentils.
- You can do it once and refrigerate it for 2-3 days. So, you can use the preparation for many snacks.

Calories: 275kcal

Lunch: *smoked salmon and avocado plate*

Ingredients

- 3 oz. smoked salmon
- 1/2 tsp mustard seeds
- 1 tsp lemon juice
- 1 tbsp chili pepper
- 1 tsp butter
- 1 tsp coriander leaves
- 1/2 avocado
- Salt and pepper to taste
- 1/2 onion
- 1/2 tomato
- 1/2 cucumber

Instructions

- In a pan, melt the tsp of butter and fry the onion and mustard seeds for about 5 minutes. The onion will take on color and become soft.
- Add the salmon, coriander leaves, a teaspoon of lemon juice, and simmer for 2-3 minutes. Remove from heat and set aside for it to cool.

- To make the salad, peel and finely slice the avocado, slice the cucumber, put them in a bowl, and scatter them with lemon juice.
- Cut the tomato, remove the seeds from the chili pepper and slice it finely.
- Place the salmon mixture in the center of a serving dish. Arrange the avocados, cucumber, and tomatoes around the salmon.

Calories: 294kcal

Snack: *Protein shake*

Ingredients

- 2 tbsp nut butter (a mix or a specific nut butter)
- 1/3 cup almond milk
- One banana, sliced
- Sweetener (optional)

Instructions

- Put fruit at the bottom of your high-speed blender.
- Then add two tablespoons of nut butter.

- Add the almond milk and, if desired, add an optional sweetener.
- Cover the blender with the lid, and blend it high for about a minute or until it's smooth. If your protein shake doesn't mix quickly, add a little more liquid and try to blend.

Advice:

You can prepare more at once and refrigerate it for 2-3 days. So, you can use the preparation for many snacks.

Calories: 298 kcal

Dinner: *Beef & Broccoli stir-fry over cauliflower rice*

Ingredients Cauliflower Rice:

- 1/4 medium onion
- 1/2 tsp of coconut oil
- 1 cup of cauliflower, cut into florets
- Salt & pepper

Beef & Broccoli Stir fry:

- 1/3 lb. thinly sliced flank steak
- 1 cup of broccoli, sliced into florets

- ❖ 1 tbsp of tamari
- ❖ 1/2 tsp of canola oil
- ❖ 1 tsp of fresh ginger, minced
- ❖ 1 garlic clove, minced
- ❖ 1/2 tsp of sesame oil
- ❖ 1/2 tsp of red pepper flakes
- ❖ 1 tsp of honey

Instructions

- For Cauliflower Rice: add the onion to the food processor or blender and mince, then add the cauliflower blossoms and process until evenly chopped.
- Heat a medium saucepan to medium-high heat. Add 1/2 teaspoon of coconut oil to the pan.
- Next, apply the mixture of the cauliflower onion — season to taste with salt & pepper.
- Sauté for 4-5 minutes, or until tender.
- Beef & Broccoli Stir: In a small bowl, add tamari, garlic clove, ginger, red pepper flakes, honey, and sesame oil. Put it aside.
- Season with salt and pepper over the flank steak

- Heat the wok or medium skillet to medium-high heat. Add the canola to the plate, then add the flank steak. Stir for 4-5 minutes until cooked through, add broccoli and tamari sauce mixture and cover.
- Stir and fry for 2 minutes.
- Serve with cauliflower rice.

Calories: 310kcal

DAY 5

Breakfast: *Omelet made with spinach and avocado, with strips of bacon*

Ingredients for omelets

- ❖ One egg, divided
- ❖ 1 tbsp water, divided
- ❖ 2 tsp unsalted butter
- ❖ 1 tbsp minced scallions, divided
- ❖ 1 tsp minced garlic, divided
- ❖ Salt and black pepper to taste

For the filling

- ❖ 2 tbsp shredded cheddar
- ❖ One strip thick-sliced bacon, cooked and chopped
- ❖ 1/2 cup fresh spinach
- ❖ 2 tbsp sliced scallions
- ❖ 2 tbsp diced tomato
- ❖ 1/3 avocado, chopped

Instructions

- For one omelet, whisk the egg and mix with a tablespoon of water and a tablespoon of minced shallot — season with salt and pepper.
- Melt two teaspoons of butter in a pan over medium heat.
- Apply the egg mixture to the skillet. Immediately, start shaking the skillet gently back and forth, stirring with tiny, rapid movements. When the eggs are set but still very moist, remove it from the fire.
- To be filled, add the cheddar, bacon, tomato, and spinach to one-half of the omelet. Fold the omelet in half and turn it to the plate; let it rest for 1 minute.

Combine sliced scallions, tomatoes, and avocados; put on top of the omelet.

Calories: 327kcal

Snack: *Granola bars with cinnamon berry*

You can see the recipe directly on the second day of the daily meal. The recipe provides a portioning of two snacks, but you can increase the doses to have snacks for several days. Keep the bars in the fridge for 3-4 days.

Lunch: *cauliflower hash browns*

Ingredients

- One egg
- 2 tbsp butter, for frying
- 1/2 tsp salt
- 1/3 yellow onion, grated
- 1/3 lb. cauliflower
- One pinch pepper

Instructions

- Rinse, trim and grate the cauliflower with the food processor or the grater.
- Put the cauliflower in a bowl. Attach the remaining ingredients and stir. Put aside for 5 to 10 minutes.
- Melt two tablespoons of butter or five teaspoons of olive oil in a no-stick pan over medium heat.
- Place the chopped cauliflower mixture in the frying pan and gently flatten it until it is around 3-4 inches in diameter.
- Fry on each side for 4-5 minutes. Change the heat and make sure they're not burning. Remember — patience is a virtue — if you flip your pancakes too fast, they can fall apart!

Calories: 316kcal

Snack: *Carrots dipped in peanut butter*

Ingredients

- 3 tbsp peanut butter
- One medium carrot, peeled

Instructions

- Chop the carrot into the sticks.
- Put the peanut butter in a small tub.
- Serve the carrot and peanut butter together. Dip the carrots in the peanut butter and use them to scoop it. Enjoy it!

Calories: 305kcal

Dinner: *Salmon, stir fry broccoli, sautéed mushrooms*

Ingredients for the Sicilian-style salmon

- One lime, juice only
- 3 oz. salmon fillet, skin removed
- 1/2 tsp dried chili flakes
- 1/2 tsp ground paprika
- 1 tsp olive oil, for drizzling
- Salt and freshly ground black pepper

For the mushrooms and broccoli

   3 oz. button mushrooms, sliced
- 2 tsp olive oil

- ❖ 1/2 garlic clove, finely chopped
- ❖ 3 oz. broccoli, chopped
- ❖ 1 tbsp chopped fresh parsley, optional

Instructions

- Preheat the oven to 350°F (180 °C).
- Place the salmon on a (lightly) greased baking sheet. Season with a teaspoon of olive oil and lime juice. Sprinkle with the chili flakes and paprika and season with salt and pepper. Bake for about 10 minutes, or until cooked through.
- Meanwhile, take a non-stick pan to heat two teaspoons of olive oil. First, add the mushrooms to sauté them (5 minutes), then the broccoli until cooked to your liking. Finally, add the garlic and sauté (1 minute), and incorporate the parsley.
- Serve directly with the salmon.

Calories: 311kcal

DAY 6

Breakfast: *Greek yoghurt layered with apples, cinnamon, and walnuts*

Ingredients

Greek Yogurt Walnut Caramel Dip

- ❖ 3/4 cup vanilla nonfat Greek yoghurt
- ❖ 1 tbsp caramel topping
- ❖ 1/2 tsp cinnamon
- ❖ 1 ½ tbsp California walnuts, chopped

Apple

- ❖ One sliced apple

Instructions

- Preheat the oven to 350 ° F (177°C). Arrange the chopped walnuts in a single layer and toast them for 5 minutes on a baking sheet. Then remove them.
- Take a bowl or a deep plate to put the yogurt and the caramel and mix them with a knife or teaspoon to rotate the caramel in the yogurt. Finish by sprinkling the yogurt with cinnamon and nuts.

- You can arrange the apple wedges around the sauce, perhaps with a squeeze of lemon, if you don't eat it immediately, to preserve them better.

Calories: 310kcal

Snack: *Yogurt smoothie with berries*

Ingredients

- ❖ 5.3 oz. (about 3/4 cup) of non-dairy yoghurt (soy or others)
- ❖ 1 cup frozen berries (raspberries, strawberries, blueberries and/or blackberries)
- ❖ 1/4 cup of cool water or almond milk
- ❖ 1/2 tsp of vanilla extract or granulated vanilla bean powder (optional)

Instructions

- Put all the ingredients in a blender, and blend until you get a smooth consistency. If necessary, you can stop to scrape the sides. Add an extra splash of water or plant-based milk to obtain your preferred density.

- Pour the mixture into a glass so you can enjoy it with a spoon or straw.

Calories: 280Kcal

Lunch: *Mediterranean lentil salad with sun-dried tomatoes and pine nuts*

Ingredients

- Two small red onions, thinly sliced
- 1/4 cup French green lentils
- One tbsp capers (in brine), drained
- One generous handfuls basil leaf, coarsely chopped
- Three tsp pine nuts, lightly toasted
- 2-3 oil-packed sun-dried tomatoes halves, chopped
- 1/2 small bunch flat-leaf parsley, coarsely chopped
- Freshly ground pepper and sea salt, to taste
- 2 tbsp freshly squeezed lemon juice from a large lemon
- Fresh parmesan shavings (optional)
- 3 tsp extra-virgin olive oil

Instructions

- Lay the lentils in a saucepan, cover with plenty of water and bring to a boil (generally, should boil the lentils with water at a ratio of 1:3). Simmer on medium heat for 25-30 minutes, until al dente. Drain the excess water and move to the bowl to cool off.
- Apply the red onion, the basil, the parsley, the capers, the toasted pine nuts, and the tomatoes to the lentil dish.
- In a small cup, mix oil, lemon juice, and a pinch of salt and pepper with which to season the lentils.
- If required, taste and add more salt or lemon juice. Serve with parmesan shaves, if needed. Enjoy it!

Calories: 330kcal

Snack: *Protein shake*

Follow the procedure already seen on the fourth day of the meal plan. You can make the protein shake directly, only once, with double doses, to use it for two snacks.

Dinner: *Veggie and bean soup with chicken*

Ingredients

- 1/4 finely chopped yellow onion
- 1 tsp olive oil
- 1/2 celery stalk, sliced
- 1/2 cup chicken broth
- 1/2 cup cooked chicken, shredded
- 1/2 carrot peeled, quartered and sliced
- 1/3 zucchini quartered and sliced
- 1 tsp parsley chopped, optional
- 2 tbsp of white beans, any variety
- 2 tbsp red kidney beans
- Salt and pepper to taste

Instructions

- Heat the olive oil in a pot. Over medium heat. Season with pepper and salt to taste and add the onion, celery and carrot. Cook, stirring periodically, for 5-6 minutes, until the vegetables are tender.
- Put the chicken broth in the pot, then bring to a simmer.

- Add the chicken, beans, and zucchini and cook for another 5-7 minutes until the zucchini is tender.
- If required, add more salt and pepper.
- Sprinkle and serve with chopped parsley.

Calories: 324 kcal

DAY 7

Breakfast: *Egg butter*

Ingredients

- One large egg
- 1 oz. butter
- 1/2 tsp sea salt
- 1/2 tsp ground black pepper
- Two seed crackers

Instructions

- Put the egg (gently) in a saucepan and cover it with cold water. Bring to a boil, even without a lid.
- Let the egg cook for about 7-8 minutes and quickly cool the egg in a basin with cold water.

- Peel the egg and chop finely. Mix with butter, pepper, and salt. Add flavorings (optional).
- Serve accompanied by two crackers. Enjoy your meal!

Calories: 311kcal

Snack: *The endomorph bread*

Ingredients

- 1/3 cup almond flour
- 2 tbsp ground psyllium husk powder
- 1/2 tsp sea salt
- 1 tsp baking powder
- 1/3 cup of water
- One egg white
- 1/2 tsp cider vinegar

Instructions

- Preheat the oven to 175°C (350°F). In a bowl, combine the dry ingredients (except the yeast).

- Meanwhile, separately, bring the water to a boil; add it and continue mixing until the liquid is completely absorbed. Add the vinegar and egg whites and continue the process for about two minutes. At this point, you can add the yeast to complete the blending. The dough must be compact.
- Remove the mixture from the bowl. Give it the shape of a ball and divide it into 2-3 balls according to the size you prefer.
- Prepare a baking tray with parchment paper (grease it a little) and place the prepared balls on it.
- Bake for about 50-55 minutes (depending on the oven's heat output) on the central rack. They are ready when, knocking the bottom of the sandwiches, you hear a dull sound.
- Let them cool. Enjoy your meal!

Calories: 288Kcal

Lunch: *Sweet potato with shredded chicken, drizzled with barbecue sauce*

Ingredients

- ❖ 2 teaspoon olive oil
- ❖ One pinch salt
- ❖ 4 oz. large sweet potato
- ❖ 1 ½ tbsp green onions, thinly sliced
- ❖ 1/2 cup red cabbage, shredded
- ❖ 1 ½ oz. rotisserie chicken breast
- ❖ 1/4 cup barbecue sauce (63 g)

Instructions

- Heat the oven up to 220°C (425° F). Line a baking sheet with thin parchment paper.
- Break the chicken breast into small pieces and set aside.
- Use a fork to make holes in the potato and move it to the pan you prepared earlier.
- Cook the potato for 40-50 minutes. You can use a toothpick/fork to check it is ready. In case, it will get punctured easily.

- Take a pan to heat the red cabbage over medium heat and add the barbecue sauce. Brown for about 3 minutes, so as to soften the cabbage.
- Add the minced chicken and mix it with the cabbage. Remove the pan from the heat.
- Remove the potato from the oven and cut it in half lengthwise. When the potato has cooled enough to be processed, collect the pulp with a spoon leaving a layer of about 6 mm.
- With the chicken and cabbage filling, fill the sweet potato skins, drizzle with barbecue sauce and garnish with sliced green onions.
- Have fun!

Calories: 308kcal

Snack: *Lentil hummus and Veggies*

Follow the procedure already seen on the fourth day of the meal plan. You can make Hummus directly, only once with, double doses, to use it for two snacks.

Dinner: *shrimp skewers with chimichurri*

Ingredients Shrimp skewers

- 5 oz. shrimp
- 1/3 lemon, juice
- 2 tsp tamari soy sauce
- 1 garlic clove, crushed
- 1/2 tsp salt
- 1 pinch chili flakes
- 1 scallion stalk

Chimichurri

- 4 tsp light olive oil
- 1 tbsp white wine vinegar
- 4 tbsp fresh parsley, finely chopped
- 1 garlic clove, finely chopped
- 1/2 red chili peppers, finely chopped
- 1/2 tsp dried oregano
- 1/2 tsp salt
- 1 pinch pepper

Instructions

- Clean the shrimp by first washing them and then removing the head, legs, and carapace, leaving the tail if you prefer. Use a small knife to remove the central vein (the intestine) by making an incision in the back.
- Take a bowl to prepare the marinade, mixing well the soy sauce, lemon juice, crushed garlic, chili flakes, and salt.
- Place the shrimp in the marinade and leave in the refrigerator for at least 15 minutes.
- Prepare the chimichurri by taking a bowl and mixing the ingredients. Leave to rest to allow the flavors to combine.
- Cut the onion stems into sticks of 2.5 cm (length).
- Take the shrimp that you have kept in the fridge and pierce them with wooden sticks (kebab style), alternating them with the green onions you have prepared (sticks).
- Prepare the barbecue or grill and cook the skewers for about 6-7 minutes until they become opaque.

- Pour the chimichurri with a spoon on the skewers, and enjoy your meal!

Advice:

It is advisable to wet the sticks before forming the skewers to prevent them from burning on the grill.

Calories: 301Kcal

CHAPTER FOUR

Simple Exercise For Your Body Type

A challenge for an endomorph is to lose weight and burn stubborn body fat. An endomorphic body is essentially the type of body that's predisposed to store body fat. Being an endomorph, it is easy to put on weight and muscle. Excess body fat shedding is the problem. The problem with lifting weights as an endomorph is that, most certainly, you build the muscle, but it's concealed by a layer of fat that never exposes the muscles in their whole. The traditional endomorph look is 'bulky.' But we want to be sliced. We're the opposite of ectomorphs in that they find it incredibly difficult to put on muscle because they have a hyperactive metabolism. Whatever muscle they put on, their body will most likely use it as fuel, in addition to storing fat.

In comparison, endomorphs have an incredibly sluggish metabolism and their sensitivity to insulin is very high. And for the mesomorph, their complete metabolism resides between the poles of endomorph and ectomorph. The roles of their body are optimized: the correct balance between anabolism and catabolism. An individual with a mesomorphic body type can be easily identified at the gym. He's the guy, or she's the girl who doesn't have to work out necessarily. They don't bust their asses on the treadmill or the escalator and get all hot and sweaty like the endomorphs, nor pump half as much iron to build some mature muscle like the ectomorph. The mesomorphs will perform well on any diet. They can easily get bulked up on a diet of high calories or shredded on low calories.

Exercise with High Intensity for Short Periods

How do you lower your body fat levels in a short period while retaining muscle tone and increasing strength? You'll need to make a few slight but important adjustments to your diet and exercise routine for successful results. To lose weight, exercise with workouts of high intensity/short length.

You will need to choose particular foods committed to elevating your metabolism and keeping you energized. You'll need to spend some time designing your personalized fat-burning program and performing your workouts based on your fitness level and lifestyle.

Fat-burning devices aren't the same as cutting calories. They're mainly concerned with stimulating the endocrine system while controlling the blood sugar levels all day long. Effectively, this is achieved by splitting the daily calories into six different meals.

Having six small meals may sound like eating a lot, but your body will find it a welcome change as nutrients circulate through your bloodstream continuously. Many who miss meals may believe they consume fewer calories, but calorie intake is just one of their metabolic processes. If you cause your blood sugar levels to drop for a prolonged period, the body needs the brain to be fed the glucose. Since the brain takes precedence over all other autonomic systems, the results or actions would be less than stellar. That is why, once they have their coffee cup or feel slow during the day before they eat their first meal, they feel fuzzy. Fat-burning diets give your body fuel to boost your metabolism, and all that nutritious food helps your exercise. The strong combination will keep you burning fat for the entire day.

Recall that everybody is different; there are variations in specific body types to remember. Many that are round (endomorphic) have trouble burning fat and have a decreased metabolism. Everybody cannot fit perfectly into the mold. Endomorphs need participation at a different level of fitness than others. Endomorphs are genetically predisposed to fat retention and are not generally involved in vigorous athletics. Their arms, heads, shoulders, stomachs, hips and legs bear their fat. Most of the coaches and gurus regarding health and well-being appear to be mesomorphs. Their body type appears to be athletic, heavily muscled and lean; they have body balance and beauty, and enjoy working out. Mesomorphs are typically athletic and broad-shouldered with a strong potential for burning fat. Few of them have had to struggle with obesity;

they seem to develop an interest in sports or other hobbies in their early lives. They quickly get it off as they gain extra weight.

To make endomorphs lose weight, exercise at first must be gradual and of low intensity. Walking is a perfect initiating practice for efficient burning of fat. The most effective way to maintain your body fat while maintaining your muscle mass is to carefully reduce your fat level by one to two pounds a week. Fat-burning exercises will drive the body's metabolism as the system transitions to its fat-burning routine for 24 hours. Don't get bullied on television by fitness models; work at your own pace and stay inspired. Fitness is like brushing your teeth; you're going to have to do it forever. The reality is, even those people who look amazing on TV need to spend a great deal of time and effort on keeping fit. One thing you need to remember in your attempt to lose weight is that workouts have to be fun and engaging to keep you going for the long term.

Endomorphs, sadly, are the ones who find it very easy to put on weight; one saying is, "we just have to look at food and put on weight." We need to work diligently to lose weight and the excess body fat that we have gained over the years. One of the key reasons for this is our slow metabolism, of course, not because we tend not to do anything at all. One approach is to use some smart and quick methods of training geared to accelerating our sluggish metabolism. We want our bodies to actively burn fat and develop lean muscles. And eventually attaining the physical body that we desired and dreamed of. It would also help if we have a common target and deadline to work towards, such as a model photo-shoot date, having our beach body by a certain date, or just for our well-being and well-being to be proud by our boyfriend, girlfriend or wife.

Smart and Simple Training Methods

One of the key concepts for us (endomorphs) is that to accelerate our bodies' metabolism, we need to be practicing at a quick practicing pace. What does that mean for us, practically?

I.   Short rest periods (10-30s) between sets

II.   Quick rest periods (30-60s) between exercises

Looks easy or challenging? Well, it depends on the way you see it, your initial fitness base, and the timing being right. If you are strict with these two easy steps, it will help you consume more energy in a shorter period and burn more calories during your workouts. You're certainly going to breathe hard and sweat from this rigorous routine, but you're certainly going to feel fantastic! It achieves the purpose of improving the metabolism of our bodies and the impact of fat-burning after work out!

Some great methods of training which take advantage of short rest periods between sets are:

I.   Super sets - Super sets are two exercises performed back and forth together. It can be either a large muscle with a small muscle or two muscles of the same class opposing each other.

II. Drop sets - Drop sets are essentially the same exercise starting with one weight and then lowering the weight to make another set again, each set being performed to fail. You determine how many drops you want to experience based on how hard you want to reach a certain muscle group. It can be achieved at the last collection of a section of the body.

III. In-set super sets - Within the same set of the same weight; this is achieved by two exercises together. A good example is the DB press of DB flies.

IV. Triple sets - 3 separate exercises back and forth together!

V. Quad sets - 4 separate exercises back and forth!

VI. Five sets - 5 separate movements back and forth!

VII. 10 sets - 10 separate movements back and forth!

VIII. Methods above require doing exercises one after another without breaks besides going to the gym or changing weights. It includes setting up your preparation, weights and equipment at a time when your local gym isn't so busy. It is certainly for more experienced bodybuilders and people who have had good training behind them for at least a year or two.

Now we can't keep this kind of training method physically forever even though we have a great diet, and the right supplements all help us recover from our workouts and develop. However, to improve this, these smart and quick training approaches can be integrated regularly every four weeks into your base program. I mean using one of the above superset training methods every four weeks for the next four weeks, then go back to your basic training program. Our bodies and mind easily adjust within 3-4 weeks to the training schedules, so we need to change our workouts every 3-4 weeks accordingly. It will strengthen your body to adapt, develop and alter, and eventually keep efficiently burning your body's metabolism! This smart and easy training method is one technique that I would recommend, and that I enjoy using myself.

For some other very simple and insightful training methods, change your workouts every 2Nd or 3rd session, and change the order of exercises that you do for each part of the body.

It will help you strike your muscles from various directions, and for the first time, you can feel your muscles being called into motion. It will keep you and your body on your toes, forcing your body to shift, alter, and develop constantly and eventually burn fat to reveal the lean muscle underneath!

Now, much of what I've shared is probably not new to you, but sometimes we need to hear it differently, even from another viewpoint, including myself. It's also different again because you've completed the most, if not all, of the above training strategies, and you can look at it again and see what this time and why it worked for you.

Work with your Genetics for Maximum Fitness Results

Did you know that great bodies come in many forms and shapes? Genetics play an enormous role in the ability of your body to achieve a certain appearance. A John Goodman would probably never achieve a physique of the style Brad Pitt, but if he does it right, he can still look good. It is essential to understand and work with your genetics, not against them. It's crucial to build reasonable expectations; otherwise, there'll be dissatisfaction, and people tend to give up when they're upset.

Knowing the nature of the body and anatomy can be very helpful. By acquiring this expertise, you can build more successful workouts by laying a framework to tweak to produce the best results possible. For example, if you are already lean and have a quick metabolism, you can get away with less aerobic exercises and concentrate more on weight training. If you're trying to lose heaviness and have a tendency to put weight on quickly, you should concentrate mainly on exercise and a more restrictive diet while using weights to retain muscle mass.

Working Out for Your Body Type

Three major types of the body exist: ectomorphs, mesomorphs, and endomorphs. Most people represent a combination of two styles of the body. Think of it as a continuum. It goes from Ecto to Meso to Endo. Everyone is dropping somewhere along the continuum but not necessarily spotting on one particular form. The way that you learn depends on what your genetics are. You will want to find out where you fit in on the spectrum; that way, you can work with your genetics in a way that works.

Ectomorphs

Ectos, also known as "hard gainers," tend to be on the shorter side and have difficulty putting muscle on. Yet they can get away with eating more without gaining weight as well. People appear to dislike ectos for being the guys who eat food without contributing to their love handles. If you're an ectomorph, you might consider yourself unfortunate as it makes it difficult to put on muscle, but in Hollywood, ectomorphs build a great camera look! Not to mention the camera increases about 10 pounds to your frame so that you'll look like a screen stud statue! Ectomorphs have to hit hard on the weights and make sure they eat enough calories to sustain muscle development. The primary emphasis should be on intense compound exercises in the 6–12 rep range. When it comes to fitness, ectomorphs ought to take caution not to overdo it. Excess cardio can eventually burn essential calories required to add muscle. If you are a genuinely healthy ecto, you need to make sure that you compensate by eating more to offset the consumed calories. For ectomorphs, walking is perfect because it is muscle-sparing. Shy away from intense exercise, since it can eat up your hard-earned muscle.

Mesomorphs (the Intermediaries)

Mesomorphs would have the easiest time to achieve a lean athletic appearance since they are formed naturally. They can put muscle on reasonably quickly while remaining lean, but they should do daily cardio bouts. Naturally, they appear to have a V-shaped torso, which lays a good foundation for a Hollywood look.

Mesomorphs find it easier to put on fat than ectomorphs, so high-intensity cardio should not be a concern. Mesos can perform almost any cardio that they like as long as they track what changes are happening in their bodies. Mesos should concentrate on improving their shape and providing meaning. Good size muscles will come reasonably soon, so exercise should be a major part of the routine, as shedding fat will show off the muscles. Also, as a side note, mesomorphs need to be careful not to overdo it in the weight room because if they are not careful, they may become too bulky.

Endomorphs

Males are going to have a round body shape while females are going to be very curvy. Endomorphs possess a dense bone structure and easily store fat. Many men you see that you might think are endomorphs are just mesomorphic but overweight. Females will certainly work to their benefit on these genes. Guys can do it too, but they'll have to closely watch their food and hit the aerobics like there's no tomorrow, none of which is fun to guys, but it's what needs to be done.

The target of endos is to strive for cleanliness. Evite the body in pear form by doing more cardio and watching what you eat. I strongly recommend a lower endomorphic carb diet, and make sure of that as diet is going to be the most important player here. For both genders with endomorphic genetics, a perfect look can be accomplished, but it requires quite a bit of practice. Stop the sushi bars all-you-can-eat, and instead go for a grilled chicken salad. Exercises should be mainly cardio-based with resistance training. But muscle and fat come very naturally for endomorphs, so having enough muscle shouldn't be a problem. That's why you're going to turn your focus and accentuate your form towards the cardio.

Don't Use your Genetics as an Excuse

Just because you've identified yourself to be an ectomorph, do not start reaching for the Cheetos. Be truthful with yourself, and regardless of your body type, your diet should always be made up of nutritious foods that will support your body. Yeah, ectos are motivated to eat more, but this does not mean reaching the McDonald's drive-through. Get two rather than just one chicken breast. The kinds of dietary practices that should be followed are these.

No matter what your biology may be, don't get discouraged. Everybody has a challenge; whether putting on muscle or losing weight, the challenges you'll have to tackle will always come in. If it were easy to achieve a Hollywood body, everyone would have one. Regardless of your biology, you will always have to invest as much time, commitment and dedication, cliché as it may sound. But you can build a better route for yourself by understanding your body type to meet your goals.

There is a misconception that endomorphs are not capable of losing body fat. Since most don't feed enough for their particular body form, this book will provide some actionable tips on endomorphic diet. You'll be sadly disappointed if you're an endomorph and you want to live like an ectomorph (naturally thin ones). Their body shape and metabolism are entirely different. You have to make some adjustments.

It is All About Synergy

The first thing to know is that it will be more difficult. While it is possible to lose fat as an endomorph, when it comes to your diet, you need to be stricter. The little routine things you do right, the better the performance will be. Eating higher protein foods, consuming more water and not skipping any meals are examples.

Beware of Carbohydrates

Carbohydrates are amongst all the macronutrients that require the most care. The user of carbs, such as a genetically slim individual or a robust individual, is a catastrophic formula. You have to eat slower-burning carbs and reduce them as well. You do not have to cut them out entirely. That's a short-term solution, and it bears a crash diet label.

Rev Up Your Metabolism

You will have to do whatever you can to accelerate your metabolism. Endomorphic metabolism is always slow and needs considerate care. Therefore, you should eat smaller meals more often than not. That will keep your metabolism in high gear. Larger meals are counterproductive.

Ignore Processed Foods

A good way to consider whether a product is good or not is the level of packaging it has. Too many processed foods will seriously hamper your growth. One example is foods that claim to be "low fat." The fat may be lower, but they often make up for it in simple sugars with carbs!

Limit Your Cheat Meals

It's good to cheat on your diet, but only if it's predetermined. Eating fast food on a whim will also take you down a slope. One cheat meal a week is perfect and helps relieve cravings. A whole cheat day should be avoided as it would set back too much of your growth.

Eat Healthy Fats

Believe it or not, certain fats are helpful for loss of weight. It's a mistake to avoid all fats because you think they're all evil. Yeah, there are poor fats like saturated and trans fats, but there are also healthy ones. They are found in foods such as eggs and salmon.

Good Body Shape

Typically, there are body shaping techniques contained in the gym environment. There are some shaping elements, but not all of the elements apply to all the women. So many shaping programs are aiming to combine the exercise of resistance with a cardiovascular or aerobic workout. Portable should be the best body shaping program — ensuring you can do them wherever and anywhere. On a more spiritual level, a target for body shaping might be to 'feel' attractive, happy and full of burning energy. This form of curriculum benefits from being particularly conducive to what body shaping is all about. Special low-impact aerobics and body shaping exercises burn calories during this intense workout and afterward.

The proper body shaping diet will decide what exercise you need to get into shape.

The nutrient breakdown effect is amplified with the supplementation of CLA (conjugated linoleic acid), which will greatly increase the body shaping results of any exercise program.

A temporary body shaping method may often result in a permanent reshaping of the body, which is extreme.

Practically all body shaping operations, except Brachioplasty, require the patient to wear a support or compression garment for two to six weeks. Men who have body shaping surgery typically undergo male breast reduction surgery to remove from their chests the sagging skin that hangs.

Plastic surgeons warn patients that surgery is not an obesity treatment. Meso-therapy is a groundbreaking modern beauty technique that acts as an alternative to conventional cosmetic work methods. On a more emotional level, a target for body shaping might be to 'feel' attractive, happy, and full of burning energy. Vibrating body shaping machines and exercise system provides tens of thousands of patients with individualized body forming facilities. And most programs struggle to do so effectively; it's very likely, particularly when the body shaping program uses bodyweight exercise concepts like a professional body shaping coach and complete body toning.

The road to "Body Shaping" opens until the pounds are gone, and the time spent in the gym pays off. Then "Body Shaping" becomes a very remote target that has a simple solution to this problem.

An important tool is the Power yoga, that has also found popularity with Hollywood movie stars and is effective for dieting, body shaping, and stress relief.

Weight Loss

For weight loss, cardiovascular health and body shaping, and aerobic exercise are important. Fitness coaching, fitness exercises, personal training, physical well-being, weight loss, and nutrition plans are all you need to read. Become a part of the most successful online body shaping and weight loss programs. I've been reading many diet and exercise books in my never-ending search to find the elusive solution to my sluggish weight-loss. The key to fruitful weight loss is a mix of long-term diet strategies and an improved workout routine. If endomorphs haven't started exercising before for weight loss, they may start with simple exercises. A licensed trainer, wellness professional, and weight-loss professional may suggest a weight loss program, weight loss exercise, weight loss diet, toning weight loss, weight loss health.

Exercise programs

Current literature suggests anaerobic exercise combined with strength building and an aerobic exercise program are the best structures to follow in workouts. People who have never exercised before should start an exercise regimen to minimize swelling, lower blood clot risks, and muscle tone. It's about what you eat with any fitness routine or discipline. Instead of focusing on your body weight, you or your friend, if you are interested in this topic for them, should focus on maintaining a healthy and balanced diet and daily exercise schedule. Be sure to visit your doctor before you undertake any workout or weight loss program.

In the following paragraphs, I will tell you about different types of physical activity that are very useful for our purpose. A note of merit, certainly, for those who follow a correct diet and carry out physical activity with good consistency, should be given the integration with CLA (conjugated linoleic acid). This has a nutrient breakdown effect that will greatly increase the body shaping results of any exercise program, as it leads our metabolism to favor the exploitation of fat as an energy source.

Aerobic exercise

Cardiovascular or aerobic exercise scans vary slightly. Some shaping programs aim to combine the exercise of resistance with a cardiovascular or aerobic workout. Current literature suggests anaerobic exercise combined with strength building and an aerobic exercise program (aerobic exercise joined with a healthy diet) can minimize body fat. This improves fatigue resistance. Examples of anaerobic exercise include running, swimming, bicycling, and cross-country skiing. Cycling, jogging, swimming and aerobic dance are examples of aerobic exercise. Burning body-fat involves aerobic exercise.

Body sculpting

Allie guides you through workouts that will give you the lean, solid body of your dreams with high-energy, high-intensity cardio and distinctive body sculpting. Perhaps better, the handles and weights are built specifically to work with the exclusive combination of aerobic and body sculpting exercises from the company. Accessible at reasonable rates are body sculpting, general wellness, workout routines, diet plans, fitness equipment and special programs to adopt. Total body sculpting combines fat-burning exercises with body-shaping movements to turn your whole body into the sleek, solid body you've always wanted. Yoga and dance-based exercises with booty movements are about sculpting the body and developing an attractive, younger-looking, curved female body form. Kickboxing and sculpting your body to the hottest tunes burn more calories than just about any other workout.

Exercise routine

Although there may be variations in natural coordination or strength capacity, they can all perform the same routine exercise. The workout routines can be nearly identical because the intended results are approximately the same. The bare midriff displays some very well-defined muscles, so it is up to a reliable role model to lead an abs-oriented exercise regimen. If you are following the real diet and exercise regimen, you can meet your goals.

Lose weight

People also fail to lose weight if the correct exercises are not performed. It explains why many people can't lose weight from some parts of their body, despite strict diets and exercise regimes. If I can only develop my flexibility as I age, then exercise and weight loss would be easier. Attach the details about the workout, and you're sure you will lose weight! Diets should be paired with weight loss exercises, or you'll never be able to lose weight.

Anaerobic exercise

It is a perfect mix of aerobic and anaerobic exercise. Current literature suggests anaerobic exercise combined with strength building and an aerobic exercise program. Anaerobic exercise needs intense muscle activity and is necessary.

Body weight

Instead of concentrating on her body weight, your wife should concentrate on keeping a healthy, balanced diet and a daily exercise schedule. Also, performing lower body and abdominal exercises twice a week and doing upper body exercises on other days. You may want to begin by doing exercises that use your body weight and do not require any specific equipment. Power Tower helps you to use your body weight as a resistance to a range of workouts to get into shape. In several cases, athletes find that their body weight starts to rise after some time without adequate exercise.

Exercise regimen

Incorporating a safe, balanced diet and the proper exercise regime will eventually allow you to get the physique you want. Cardiovascular routines work out your discipline, dedication, objectives and target exercise routine, or even frequency, length and intensity of workouts are critical for sustained results! The findings will be assumed to be lasting as long as the patient adheres to a proper diet and exercise regime.

Personal trainer

An ambassador personal fitness trainer with 20 years of health and workout experience, via support and wellness experience, will keep you going towards your goals by maintaining a strong, sincere concern for your improvement in exercise. A personal trainer will help you achieve optimal fitness benefits, adjusting your workout for your health and body goals.

Effective exercise

For any part of the body, this is a comprehensive and successful workout. This experience helps develop highly efficient workout plans for minimizing time and resources and improving performance. Pilates is a gentle, efficient exercise method, frequently involving the use of a floor mat or equipment.

Exercise programs

This experience helps develop highly efficient workout plans for minimizing time and resources and improving performance. Learn why 90% of diets, fitness plans, and supplements don't work and fix them. The concept is too often confused with other types of workout programs that are not conducive to firming and shaping.

Future gym exercise

When you are sculpted into a beautiful form, Potential Gym workout tackles all the trouble areas like the chest, shoulders, waist and back. It makes exercising at Future Gym a better alternative for therapy recovery. Exercising Potential Gym is a perfect option for a lifetime of physical health.

Exercise equipment

No fad diets, costly sports equipment or dangerous plastic surgery! My favorite fat-burning workout device, the elliptical trainer, isn't exactly amazing. Unlike most, home exercise rowing equipment works and tones the whole body!

Dance moves

Instead of gym workouts, each workout is based entirely on belly dance steps. It uses dance steps solely from the belly —

no crunches or aerobic workouts. Instead of doing some gym drills, you choose workouts that focus solely on belly dance steps.

Physical activities

Women who were exercising for body shaping purposes reported taking part in higher-intensity physical activities. Within a month or two, after the soreness has subsided, they resume exercise and normal physical activities.

The endomorph workout

If you hold most of your fat in your face (especially your neck and cheeks), around your waist, hips, and thighs, you are the classic endomorph. You're easily mistaken for a mesomorphic type of body when you're lean and healthy.

The tell-tale fat accumulation under the chin and the cheeks start showing off if you slack off working out and dieting. Since this type of body stores calories very effectively, they are much less effective at losing weight. Naturally, their metabolic rate is slower than most, making it much harder to achieve results while working out or dieting.

The classic endomorph, around the mid-portion, would have a naturally high degree of body fat. Typically, they take a pear shape or pattern. Endomorphs that are overweight will have a hard time managing their weight (think of Oprah Winfrey or John Goodman).

The abundance of fast-food restaurants and other comfort foods makes healthy living difficult for you, and you're likely to gain weight by eating less due to your natural propensity to miss meals while worried or distracted!

Classic endomorphs aren't really big fans of working out, although they may enjoy watching sports or playing them in a videogame. Since this type of body is less likely to participate in athletic events, they must exercise every day. Unlike the mesomorph or ectomorph who can get away with slacking off for a few days, after a few days off, endomorphs can quickly find their bodies slowing down and succumbing to exhaustion or tiredness.

I belabor this point because while endomorphs at their optimum bodyweight appear to be very physically attractive, they will look and feel dramatically different when they let their fat percentage go past 25-30 percent.

The Endomorph Workout

If you hate cardio, then sign up for a burial plot right now. High-intensity aerobic exercises on a short duration will save your life. Cardio routines such as rope skipping, rebounding, punching, elliptical machines or cycling. Stop swimming and aerobics with heavy effects. Since it's gentle on the body and good for the heart, you'll enjoy swimming, but it'll do nothing to help you lose weight. If you are out of shape already, you would hate high-impact aerobics. It will initially leave you feeling exhausted, and that alone will scare most endomorphs out of shape.

Hold down on the exercise for 20-30 minutes. The main secret that will be capitalizing on your asset is to improve your metabolism. Endomorphs develop muscle with the same ease as mesomorphs.

Muscle Building Workout

The truth is, many endomorphs tend to diet first and lose muscle mass rather than fat. The weight gets decrease while the metabolism gets slower. When their diet is turned back to the old way, the fat reserves become even bigger, and the muscles are still sluggish. I suggest compound workouts for at least the first six weeks if you are getting back into shape. Squats, deadlifts and chest press are the three best combination exercises for your overall body growth as an endomorph. Act to strengthen the muscles for strength training with these three exercises for high 10-12 reps and low sets (1-3). You have to pick a weight that allows you to finish your sets with proper shape and push you over the six-week training to gradually raise the weight.

Stick to a lower-carb diet rich in protein, which fully eliminates refined flour, sugar and hydrogenated fats and oils. Take fruit, vegetable and carbohydrates and, for now, avoid pasta or other refined starches. You're trying to feed the muscles for six weeks, to get them to burn fat 24/7.

CHAPTER FIVE

Healthy Eating Habits

Identifying which form of body you belong to can be empowering. It will help you better understand your body composition, the muscle-gaining activities you need to put in, the exercises that will benefit you, the foods that will help you stay healthy and lose weight, etc. Genetics will still be a step ahead of some people, no matter how hard they try. When it comes to exercise or weight loss, you can't beat your body type. Healthy eating is an important aspect of fitness, no matter your build. By recognizing your body type and knowing how to eat to make it ideal, you can improve your health and weight loss and eliminate obstacles.

Our type of body not only determines how we look but also provides information about how our body is reacting to food intake. It also defines the hormonal and sympathetic nervous system (SNS) characteristics. It has also been established that a person's body type may also determine their metabolic capabilities and differentiate them from other individuals when processing various food and weight gain or loss. That means it's a significant consideration for achieving your health goals. Most people may look like they have features in more than one of these types, but that's mostly due to the years of preparation and physical care they put into their health and body. And perhaps because of their origin, they may be a combination of two different types of bodies.

Let's get into what these types of body mean in each case and the optimal diet:

1. Ectomorph

These categories of people are slim and thin, meaning they have thin limbs and a narrow, slender body. They have a high metabolic rate that makes them immune to gaining weight but having trouble putting muscle on. Ectomorphs can get away from consuming unhealthy quantities of food without adding weight, and often have no weight loss issues. Of course, they have low body fat. But that's not to suggest they don't have to work out or live a healthy lifestyle; we all do.

What to Eat

If you belong to the group ectomorph, you must strive for higher carbohydrates and lower fats. Carbohydrates function, especially for this body type. Proteins still need to be ingested but in small amounts. Consumed fats should be of high quality.

Nuts, avocado, chia seeds, extra virgin olive oil, and coconut oil are examples. For ectomorphs, it has been proposed by some experts that 55% carbohydrates, 25% protein and 20% fats are best distributed in these proportions.

2. Endomorph

Endomorphs often believe they're the unfortunate type of body; being one of them, I always find it difficult to get results, and it seems we often have to work harder than the other two types of body to get modest results. Endomorphs are also larger, more rounded and appear to store a lot of fat. Our body shape is round and we have long joints. We have a large bone structure and some people in this group often find leading an active lifestyle a little more difficult. It may be due to the struggles and difficulties of not having the results they want like the other body types.

Our metabolic rate is characteristically very low as endomorphs, which encourages fat accumulation and the tendency to gain extra weight. For people with this type of body, this can be intimidating and exhausting, and it is understandable that some get fed-up and become lazy. But that's not the right response either; once they develop a strategy that involves knowing their form of the body, it's easier to achieve results and overall success in weight loss and fitness.

Knowing your body type will remove all the uncertainty and misinformation, and frustration. No diet or regulated eating habits will offer the success that our body types can learn and recognize. Eat for that type of body, and exercise for that type of body.

What to Eat

An endomorph will need to eat high-quality protein and fats. As far as carbohydrate intake is concerned, it is difficult but very doable for endomorphs to focus on healthy fats and proteins while adding some good low glycemic carbohydrates.

Thus, a breakdown of 25% starch, 35% protein and 40% fat. Simply put, considering the consumption of more fats and protein and fewer carbohydrates is a great place to start and, based on the results, refining may be essential.

3. Mesomorph

This form of the body is called genetically modified. Mesomorphs are lean, muscular, athletic and competitive in nature, making them excellent in sport. Their bodies are constructed proportionally, with a medium-sized bone structure and considerably lean mass. People who belong to this type of body can easily gain weight by changing their diet and activity level. Mesomorphs can quickly build muscle due to high testosterone.

What to Eat

If you're a mesomorph, consider having a healthy diet. That means the eating proportions are divided into 40% carbohydrates, 30% protein and 30% fat. The desire to quickly add muscle and weight means you can concentrate your entire life on good weight loss.

Going on a journey without a map or instructions is the same as not understanding your body type but expecting weight loss results and health improvements. Sometimes, we don't know what our body is doing to us without asking until it stops doing it. It is simple to get fit, lose weight and achieve wellness, but not easy to do. But by knowing the topic, which is our body, we can make it simpler and easier. We will have the knowledge this way, grasp the needs and get to the edge of what we want.

Healthy Eating with Low Carb Approach

Before making any drastic changes to your carbohydrate and protein intakes, be sure to always consult with your doctor to find out if this form of diet is correct for you. It is particularly important if you're having liver and kidney problems right now. The explanation for this is simple: following a high

protein diet low in carbohydrates can cause more damage to your health, particularly with low water consumption.

It is a very powerful temporary eating technique for people with an endomorphic, dominant type of body. Since most endomorphs are responsive to carbohydrates, their blood sugar increases when they eat too many calories from this food and there is a significant release of insulin by the pancreas into the bloodstream.

By removing the glucagon, this increases fat accumulation and reduces the degradation and burning of the energy of stored body fat. The glucose is released steadily into the bloodstream by using a low-carb diet, and insulin and glucagon function effectively, each doing the job properly. There is the effective delivery of nutrients through insulin, and the glucagon allows the organism to consume more energy for body fat.

By using a 40-35-25 nutrient ratio, 40% of your calories come from carbohydrates, 35% from protein and 25% from dietary fat; this is the best place to start your low-carb diet. You may also use a 40-40-20 nutrient mix, where 40% of your calories come from carbohydrates, 40% protein and 20% dietary fat.

You will lose more weight with the 40-40-20 nutrient ratio since the protein increase will burn more calories, as the protein has a higher thermic effect. When you have selected the nutrients ratio you will be using, take your daily intake of calories and use these new nutrient ratios to make your calculations. Then break them up into four equal meals once this is finished.

The easiest way to use this method is to eat your meals for a week with these low carbon nutrient ratios and then bring them up to a week's nutrient maintenance ratios.

This 10 percent reduction in your carbohydrate consumption for a week is enough to produce outstanding results without you having a significant drop in energy levels. It is how to easily lose weight while still providing the body with the everyday energy source!

It is significant because you will need high energy levels to keep exercising during weight loss. Replacing exercise with incredibly high protein is never a good choice. Note that your target is to burn off much of your aerobic body fat while using weight training to preserve your muscle.

How Many Carbs to Eat

Carbohydrates are also described as food villains. This form of food has been blamed on everything from a bloated tummy to poor moods and skin. Anyone who desires to lose weight knows that cutting back on 'starchy' carbohydrates will help with weight loss, but at the same time, there are so many theories and stories about what carbohydrates mean to lose weight and how they can be cut down, that a dietitian may become confused. However, as most dieticians and other experts suggest, carbohydrates take up 50% to 60% of all calories eaten, so information about the best form of carbs to eat is crucial.

A lot of dieters have been told in the past to eat plenty of carbohydrates. They have been seen as 'safe.' Potatoes, pasta and rice have been something you should be eating daily. The modern diet indicates that carbohydrates can be split into two distinct forms.

Simple Carbohydrates: The body digests them easily. Simple carbohydrates include refined sugars and low vitamins and minerals (although fruits are simple and include plenty of vitamins), products like fruit juice, yogurt, honey and, naturally, sugar are all simple carbohydrates.

Complex Carbohydrates: They take longer to digest and typically have many fibers and minerals in them. Vegetables, bread, cereals, wholewheat, rice, and pasta.

Modern dietary advice suggests that consuming large quantities of simple carbohydrates should not be permitted. As these types of carbs are easy to use and typically taste fine, they are used in more fast-food items. Yes, a bowl of sweetened breakfast cereal, a break with sweetened coffee and biscuits, and coke with a white bread sandwich, then tea chips and burgers mean you'd be eating just too many carbohydrates.

Looking closely at the tilt, you can see that there are very few complex carbohydrates there, too. Most of the carbohydrates consumed are simple: sugar, white bread and (simple) milk. Then a significant amount of refined sugar intake is associated with an elevated risk of diabetes and heart disease, not to mention obesity and indigestion.

Also, the complex carbs have some mud slung in them, and a common myth is that after 6 pm, no carbohydrates should be consumed (or at night, or after a five-mile pleasant run - there is no clear theory). This only works for people who would either be actively feeding or not complex carbs.

Eating a complex carbohydrate like pasta for a late dinner does not trigger any issues unless eaten with many fats.

Bodybuilding circles have also seen a lot of debate regarding how many carbohydrates it is best to consume. Carbohydrates are a required fuel for the body in general, and no health expert can rule them out. Most experts will suggest a daily ratio of 50/30/20 carbs/protein/fat. The precise number of calories you can consume on carbohydrates is down to your BMR. But bodybuilding also knows that endomorphic (those who run to fat faster than others) should be more conservative on their carb consumption than other forms of bodies. They may want to try a 40/40/20 diet or even a 40/45/15 diet. However, complex carbohydrates are usually appropriate for anyone to eat, and at any time, as long as they are part of a calorie-controlled diet, backed up by regular exercise. A healthy diet will still cut back on easy carbohydrates, including sugar, which is the real challenge for weight loss.

How to Eat

Are you an Endomorph? You are an endomorph if you happen to be rounded, medium to large-boned, short-limbed, and difficult to take-off. Very few people are true to one body form, so whether you are apple-shaped (bearing more weight in your upper body with a small back and shapely legs) or pear-shaped (slim shoulders tapering to broad hips), you have more than a hint of endomorph around you.

An extra reason to act, for an endomorph woman that has the apple form, is that excess fat borne on the upper body is the most harmful to your wellbeing. If you plan on living a long and safe life, you must get rid of it.

Just walking past a plate of delicate little pink iced cakes may seem to make you pile on weight as an endomorph. Carbs are not the best friend of an endomorph. Although simple carbs such as sugar and highly processed foods, soaked in saturated fat, would do no good at all to any somatotype (body type), unfortunately, complex carbs are not among the best endomorphic food choices.

A moderate to great protein diet with low to moderate intakes of carb can only do well. Know your protein needs to be lean. Suppose you want to lose weight and get fit to forget the lardy bacon and eggs, eat most of your carbohydrates in the first half of the day, including the late afternoon and evening high protein meals. Never miss a balanced protein meal, complex carbs and, mostly, unsaturated fats.

We have to learn to enjoy the cardio in terms of exercise. The cardio will get our fat burning with our naturally sluggish metabolism. You may prefer consistent long-distance fitness, or you may be factoring in some high-intensity aerobic exercise, but the shorter the workout, the more effort you will have to make to achieve worthwhile results.

You'll probably need some strength training to strengthen your muscles anyway.

To sharpen your form with some lean or mass muscles, you need moderate to hard resistance training with relatively short breaks between sets of rests.

Get yourself as polished as you can about endomorphic body shape, diet and exercise. You may become incredibly dissatisfied with the "one size fits all" standard systems that don't suit your personal needs.

There comes a human body in all shapes and sizes. There are quite a few styles of the body out there. For example, people with pear-shaped bodies have characteristically broad hips and slim upper bodies. On the other side, individuals with apple-shaped bodies appear to have large upper bodies and slimmer legs. Both pear-shaped and apple-shaped body forms fall under the category of an endomorph as they both have a rounded and wide look.

Of course, it isn't all about appearance. You're often called an endomorph if you pile on weight very quickly. This is particularly true when you do not get enough exercise. Endomorphs, however, often possess the capacity to bulk up rapidly while leading active lifestyles. Unfortunately, people who are born with an endomorphic body type typically have trouble losing weight. However, that doesn't mean to say that there's nothing an endomorph can do to change their physique. When one follows an endomorphic diet, there are a variety of things to bear in mind.

Here are some tips for a healthy endomorphic diet:

- ❖ Take care of the carbohydrates you eat - If you're very serious about weight loss, then you need to look at your carbohydrate intake. One cannot emphasize enough the importance of concentrating on this part of your diet. It is important to note that your body's metabolism does not process carbs like a naturally slim individual. It would help if you were sure to restrict the carbohydrate intake to prevent issues. That doesn't mean you need to take it out of your diet entirely, though. Your body also needs a big macronutrient, after all. Only make sure you eat carbs that burn slower.

- ❖ Stay away from processed products – It's no secret that eating too many processed foods isn't a healthy diet. Doing so would more than likely interfere with your growth and dramatically set you back. Don't be misled by the alleged health advantages these food forms offer. E.g. many of them claim to be low in fat but filled with simple quick-burning sugars.
- ❖ Be sure you eat healthy fats only - It is a common misconception among endomorphic dietitians that all fat types are bad for you. That isn't the case however.

Staying away from all of the fats together based on this common theory will better benefit your ill diet. Although trans fats and saturated fats are deemed bad for your health, there are still healthy fat types for you. Eggs and salmon constitute a decent source of healthy fats. Make sure you get enough of your food.

Nurturing a Healthy Culture

The modern-day workplace is an atmosphere far different from the one in which our parents worked. However, one aspect remains unchanged—human body's inner workings. Currently, not much in the human body has evolved since prehistoric times. It helps us understand why lifestyles today can be so harmful to our overall health and wellbeing. Rewind to the roots of our cavemen...their bodies released adrenaline in a fight or flight reaction to the potential threat from vicious predators. When we deal with the relentless intensity of corporate life, we release adrenalin. The stress will result in possible burnout. Cavemen must have been looking for food; when they ate, insulin released from their body to regulate their sugar levels and store any surplus as fat because their bodies didn't know when the next meal was coming. Fast forward into our diet today...our bodies are bombarded with refined sugars, which cause blood sugars to soar. Our bodies have to protect themselves by releasing large amounts of insulin to 'mop up' the carbohydrates, converted to fat. Continuing this method results in excessive weight gain. More significantly, our bodies gradually relinquish their attempts to protect themselves against the threat of sugar snacks and insulin resistance that can lead to diabetes.

But what will resilient leaders do to motivate workers to eat a balanced and nutritious diet?

Action 1: Break down Food Theories. Let people know that eating healthy is a lifestyle that needs to be practiced for a lifetime, not a sacrificial practice to achieve weight loss in the short term. It is also important for people to recognize that their body shapes vary based on the genes they inherit. There are three main forms of the body (ectomorphs, endomorphs, and mesomorphs), and these should be considered when setting targets for weight loss and when deciding on suitable exercise activity. Muhammad Ali, for example, probably wouldn't have excelled in the 60-meter hurdles.

Typical endomorphic characteristics: soft and round body, absorbs muscle and fat very quickly, usually short and stormy, round mechanics, find fat and sluggish metabolism hard to lose.

Typical mesomorphic features: athletic, hard body with well-defined muscles, rectangular body, solid, gain muscle easily and gain more fat easily than ectomorphs.

Typical characteristics of an ectomorph: compact fragile frame and bone structure, lean muscle mass, weight gain, and possess low high metabolism.

Action 2: Help others understand the possible danger of consuming a diet filled with processed sugars and carbohydrates (such as fizzy soft drinks, muffins, white bread, etc.). Increase understanding of foods with a low 'Glycemic Load' containing slower carbohydrate releases and help regulate blood sugar levels.

Action 3: When people become more appreciative of their food and how full it makes them feel, good eating habits grow. A 'hunger scale' poster in the canteen area will help workers eat more when needed (a 'hunger scale' allows people to decide how hungry they are on a scale from one to ten, with 1 'feeling hungry' and 10 'not hungry at all).

Action 4: Breakfast king. Everybody seems to be joining in on the fact that having breakfast is a good idea, but it seems like very few people have time. How does your organization get employees on the right foot to start their working day? One approach will be to have a microwave to make porridge when they arrive in the morning if they wish.

Action 5: Encourage people to carry snacks in between mid-morning and mid-afternoon. Study how convenient it is for workers to access snack foods with a balanced mix of gradual carbohydrate release, protein and healthier fats. Such a snack may be a small piece of fruit and a sprinkle of pumpkin seeds and almonds. Not all fruits are the same when it comes to regulating blood sugars—bananas and grapes are the worst offenders; however, berries contain the slower release of xylose sugar that has a much lower glycemic load.

Action 6: Many people understand the need to drink plenty of water during the day at regular intervals, but very few do. The sensation of hunger can often be simply due to a lack of daily fluids. It can be very normal in long meetings where a break occasion generally sees people drinking tea or coffee cups rather than their bodies' water. Lack of water in the body can also be misinterpreted as hunger, urging colleagues to drink a glass of water, waiting seven minutes and then testing how hungry they are.

Action 7: Why does it take sugar sweets, milk chocolate snacks, or muffins for the meetings' energy conservation choices? Several healthier options can provide a longer, more stable energy source without sending blood sugar through the roof. Why not launch 'Fruity Fridays' daily, and inspire people to consider alternative healthy snacks?

Action 8: Public displays of a person's weight will put people off taking part in a program, so consider an alternative measure such as a figure for 'absolute circumference measurements.' It is calculated simply by adding the circumferences of the abdomen, back, thigh, and upper arm together.

Eating Right to Gain Muscles

If you want to build muscles, you should have a good diet for proper muscle building and regular weightlifting exercises. The maximum benefits of your exercises and muscle-building program can only be provided through an appropriate diet. Your muscle fibers will undergo constant weight lifting and other aerobic exercises. Thus, the only way you can compensate for this dilemma is by careful diet plans to help regenerate muscle fibers stronger and larger than ever.

You should know your body type before you schedule a diet to build your muscle. It is mostly three distinct types. It is really important to eat more calories in your diet because calories will help repair and promote muscle cell growth. But instead of unhealthy processed foods, select good quality calories. Don't suck up more calories if you're a mesomorph and plan to lose a few pounds. Thoroughly study your body type and add calories your muscles need.

Good food is the true hero that will make your muscles grow stronger and healthier than ever.

Choose from the meal menu that provides 2 to 2.4 grams of protein per kg of body weight per day. More protein intakes are recommended for ectomorphs and endomorphs. Even consuming rich protein sources such as chicken, fish, milk and egg, olive oil, and nuts are good for substantial healthy fat content. Carbohydrates will benefit you a great deal too. When preparing a diet for muscle building, you can never miss breakfast as it is one of the essential meals for beautifully formed muscles.

When you miss it, it can also hamper your fitness as well as your healthy muscle-building regime. Increase your meal frequency from 3 to 5 or 6 daily to work harder on your body's metabolism levels.

Stick lots of water into your diet. Water is the vital agent that helps metabolize meals and muscle-building processes in your intestines. Drink two to four liters of water a day instead of alcohol and soft drinks that contain non-nutritional calories and unhealthy content of sugars. By adding protein powder into your diet, you can meet your muscle-building goals. There are several thousand claiming to create muscles by intaking safe protein supplements.

CHAPTER SIX

Endomorph Recipes

Cauliflower Tots

Ingredients

- ❖ Cooking spray
- ❖ 2 tbsp. Sriracha
- ❖ 1 large egg, lightly beaten
- ❖ 1 c. shredded cheddar
- ❖ 1 c. freshly grated Parmesan
- ❖ 2/3 c. panko breadcrumbs
- ❖ 2 tbsp. Freshly chopped chives
- ❖ 4 Cauliflower florets, steamed
- ❖ Kosher salt
- ❖ Freshly ground black pepper
- ❖ 1/2 c. ketchup

Instructions For Oven

- Preheat to 375°Fahrenheit. Grease cooking spray on a large baking sheet.
- Beat steamed cauliflower into a food processor until riced. Place riced cauliflower onto a clean kitchen towel and squeeze water to drain.
- Move cauliflower with cheese, cheddar, parmesan, panko, and chives to a large bowl and blend until mixed. To fry, season with salt and pepper.
- Take 1 tablespoon of mixture and roll it with your hands in a tater-tot shape. Place it on the ready baking sheet and bake until the tots are golden for 15 to 20 minutes.
- Meanwhile, make spicy ketchup: In a small serving bowl, mix ketchup and Sriracha and blend.
- Serve soft tots of cauliflower with spicy ketchup.

For Air Fryer

- Beat steamed cauliflower into a food processor until riced. Place riced cauliflower onto a clean kitchen towel and squeeze water to drain.

- Move cauliflower with cheese, cheddar, parmesan, panko, and chives to a large bowl and blend until mixed. To try, season with salt and pepper.
- Take 1 tablespoon of mixture and roll it with your hands in a tater-tot shape. Working in lots, place in a single layer of air fryer basket and cook for 10 minutes at 375 °F until tots are golden.
- Meanwhile, make spicy ketchup: In a small serving bowl, mix ketchup and Sriracha and blend.
- Serve soft tots of cauliflower with hot ketchup.

Servings: 4

Brussels Sprout Chips

Ingredients

- 1 tbsp. extra-virgin olive oil
- 1/2 lb. Brussels sprouts, thinly sliced
- 1 tsp. garlic powder
- Kosher salt
- 2 tbsp. freshly grated parmesan, plus more for garnish
- Freshly ground black pepper

❖ Caesar dressing, for dipping

Instructions For Oven

- Preheat oven to 375°Fahrenheit. Toss brussels sprouts with oil, parmesan and garlic powder in a large bowl, and seasoning with salt and pepper. Spread over a medium baking sheet in an even layer.
- Bake for 10 minutes, toss, and bake for another 8 to 10 minutes, until golden and crisp. Garnish with more parmesan and serve dipping with Caesar dressing.

For Air Fryer

- Toss brussels sprouts with oil, parmesan and garlic powder in a large bowl and season with salt and pepper. Arrange in the air fryer in one even sheet.
- Bake at 350°F for 8 minutes, toss and bake for an additional 8 minutes, until golden and crisp.
- Garnish with more parmesan and serve dipping with Caesar dressing.

Servings: 2

Bacon Avocado Fries

Ingredients

- 24 thin strips of bacon
- 3 avocados
- 1/4 c. ranch dressing, for serving

Instructions For Oven

- Preheat oven to 425°Fahrenheit. Slice each avocado into 8 wedges of equal size. Wrap each wedge in bacon, and cut bacon if necessary. Place them on a baking sheet, seam side down.
- Bake for 12 to 15 minutes until the bacon is cooked through and crispy.
- Use ranch dressing to eat.

For Air Fryer

- Slice each avocado into 8 wedges of equal size. Wrap each wedge with a bacon strip, and cut bacon if necessary.
- Place a single layer in the air fryer tray. Cook for 8 minutes at 400°F until the bacon is cooked and crispy.

- With ranch dressing, serve wet.

Servings: 4

Smashed Broccoli

Ingredients

- ❖ Kosher salt
- ❖ Crushed red pepper, for serving
- ❖ Extra-virgin olive oil, for frying
- ❖ 2 garlic cloves, smashed
- ❖ Lemon wedges, for serving
- ❖ 1 c. grated Parmesan
- ❖ Flaky sea salt, for serving
- ❖ 1 large head broccoli, cut into florets

Instructions For Oven

- Blanch the broccoli in salted water until they turn bright green. Drain them and immediately pass them in cold water. Drain the broccoli again and pat dry with paper towels.
- On a clean work surface, use the bottom of a glass cup to mash the broccoli without letting it fall apart.

- In a large pan over medium heat, pour enough olive oil to cover the bottom of the pan, add the garlic and let it sauté for 2 minutes. Remove the garlic from the pan.
- Add the broccoli in an even layer and cook without moving until the bottom of the broccoli is crisp and golden. Turn and cook until crisp on the other side as well.
- Remove the broccoli from the pan and transfer it to a paper towel-lined plate to drain. Work in batches to cook the remaining broccoli.
- Season the broccoli with lemon juice, parmesan, flaked sea salt and red pepper flakes.

Servings: 2

Kung Pao Brussels Sprouts

Ingredients

- 2 cloves garlic, minced
- 2 lb. brussels sprouts, halved
- 2 tbsp. extra-virgin olive oil
- Kosher salt

- 1 tbsp. cornstarch
- Freshly ground black pepper
- 1 tbsp. sesame oil
- 1/2 c. water
- 1/2 c. low-sodium soy sauce
- 2 tsp. apple cider vinegar
- 1 tbsp. hoisin sauce
- 1 tbsp. packed brown sugar
- 2 tsp. garlic chili sauce
- Pinch crushed red pepper flakes
- Sesame seeds, for garnish
- Green onions, thinly sliced, for garnish
- Chopped roasted peanuts, for garnish

Instructions

- Preheat oven to 425°Fahrenheit. Toss Brussels, cut in half lengthwise, with olive oil on a large rimmed baking sheet and season with salt and pepper.
- Bake until brussels sprouts tenderly and slightly crispy until brussels sprouts, about 20 minutes. Transfer sprouts from brussels to a large bowl.
- Heat sesame oil in a minor skillet, over medium heat. Add garlic and cook for around 1 minute until it is

fragrant. Add soy sauce, water, vinegar, hoisin sauce, brown sugar and chili paste for garlic. Bring the mixture to a boil, then lessen the heat and simmer for around 3 minutes, until thickened.
- Pour sauce over the sprouts in brussels and mix to through. Return brussels sprouts to a baking sheet and broil until glazed and sticky brussels sprouts.
- Until serving, garnish it with peanuts, sesame seeds and green onions.

Servings: 2

Cool Ranch Zucchini Chips

Ingredients
- Cooking spray
- 2 zucchinis, sliced very thinly into coins
- 1 tbsp. extra-virgin olive oil (for baked version only)
- 1 tbsp. ranch seasoning
- 1 tsp. dried oregano
- Kosher salt
- Freshly ground black pepper

Instructions For Oven

- Preheat oven to 225°C. Grease cooking spray on a large baking sheet. Cut the zucchini into very thin pieces. Tap courgettes with paper towels for removing excess moisture.
- Toss the zucchini with oil in a wide bowl, then toss into ranch seasoning, oregano, salt, and pepper. Place onto baking sheets in a single layer.
- Bake for about 1hr and 20 minutes until crispy. Before serving, allow cooling to room temperature.

For Air Fryer

- Slightly grease air sprinkler basket with cooking spray. Slice the zucchini into very thin pieces. Tap courgettes with paper towels for removing excess moisture.
- Toss zucchini in a wide bowl, seasoning with ranch, oregano, salt, and pepper. Place the basket in a single layer (a little overlap is OK!).
- Air fry for 6 minutes at 375°F, then turn over and cook for another 6 minutes. Remove the golden chips and continue to cook the remaining chips until

golden and crispy, 2 to 4 minutes, shaking basket in each minute to allow even crisping.

Servings: 4

Bang Cauliflower

Ingredients

- ❖ 2 tbsp. sweet chili sauce
- ❖ 3 tbsp. extra-virgin olive oil
- ❖ 1 tsp. chopped cilantro, for garnish
- ❖ Juice of 1 lime
- ❖ 1 medium cauliflower, cut into florets
- ❖ 3 cloves garlic, minced
- ❖ kosher salt
- ❖ 1 tbsp. sriracha
- ❖ Freshly ground black pepper

Instructions For Oven

- Preheat oven to 425°Fahrenheit. Whisk olive oil, sweet chili sauce, Sriracha, lime juice, and garlic together in a small cup.

- Toss the cauliflower in sauce on a broad baking sheet until thoroughly coated. Sprinkle with salt and pepper. Spread over an even layer and roast, for 30 to 35 minutes, until slightly golden and soft. Garnish, and serve with cilantro.

For Air Fryer

- Whisk olive oil, sweet chili sauce, Sriracha, lime juice, and garlic together in a large cup.
- Put the cauliflower in the cup, season generously with salt and pepper, and mix well to combine.
- In the Air Fryer bowl, put a third of the cauliflower in a single layer. Cook for 12 minutes at 360°F, then toss halfway.

Servings: 6-8

Garlic-Parm Zucchini Sauté

Ingredients

- ❖ 2 cloves garlic, minced
- ❖ 3 large zucchinis, cut into rounds
- ❖ 1/2 tsp. dried oregano

- ❖ Pinch of crushed red pepper flakes
- ❖ Kosher salt
- ❖ Freshly ground black pepper
- ❖ 1 tbsp. extra-virgin olive oil
- ❖ 1/4 c. freshly grated Parmesan

Instructions

- Heat oil in a large saucepan over medium heat. Add garlic, and cook for 30sec, until fragrant. Connect oregano and zucchini. Cook for about 10 minutes, until the zucchini is tender. Season with salt, pepper and a small flake of red pepper.
- Serve warmly and top with parmesan.

Servings: 4

Perfect Mashed Cauliflower

Ingredients

- ❖ 2 medium heads cauliflower, florets removed
- ❖ 6 oz. cream cheese softened
- ❖ 1/3 c. milk
- ❖ Kosher salt

- ❖ Freshly ground black pepper
- ❖ Freshly chopped chives, for garnish
- ❖ Butter, for serving

Instructions

- Hold a big saucepan of water to boil. Append the cauliflower florets and cook for 10 minutes until soft. Drain well, press paper towels to extract the excess water as much as possible.
- Return to the pot and mash cauliflower with a potato masher until the chunks remain smooth and not big.
- Incorporate cream cheese and milk, season with salt and pepper and mash until thoroughly mixed and smooth. (Add a few spoons of more milk before target consistency is reached).
- Season with more pepper, garnish with chives and finish with a butter pat.

Servings: 4

Roasted Broccolini

Ingredients

- ❖ 1 lb. Broccolini
- ❖ 2 tbsp. extra-virgin olive oil
- ❖ Kosher salt
- ❖ Freshly ground black pepper
- ❖ Crushed red pepper flakes

Instructions

- Preheat oven to 425°Fahrenheit. Place the broccolini and drizzle with oil on a large baking sheet. Season to coat with salt, pepper and a sprinkle of red pepper flakes.
- Roast slightly for 30 minutes, until fork-tender and ends are charred.

Servings: 1

Sun-Dried Tomatoes

Ingredients

- ❖ 2 pints cherry tomatoes, halved
- ❖ 1 tbsp. extra-virgin olive oil

- ❖ 1 tsp. dried oregano (optional)
- ❖ Kosher salt
- ❖ Freshly ground black pepper

Instructions

- Heat the oven to 225 degree celsius, and line a broad parchment paper baking sheet. Combine tomatoes with oil and oregano in a wide bowl, then season with salt and pepper if necessary.
- Arrange tomatoes on a baking sheet which are cut side up. Roast for 45 minutes to 2 hours, until fully dry.

Servings: 2

Cauliflower Rice

Ingredients

- ❖ Kosher salt
- ❖ 2 tbsp. extra-virgin olive oil
- ❖ 1 tbsp. freshly chopped rosemary
- ❖ 1 tsp. fresh thyme leaves
- ❖ Freshly ground black pepper

- 2 tbsp. freshly chopped parsley
- 1 large head cauliflower, cut into florets

Instructions

- Place florets in a large food processor and pulse until finely chopped, or grate florets around the medium holes with a box grater.
- Put riced cauliflower in a clean kitchen towel to remove any excess moisture.
- Heat oil in a big saucepan above medium heat. Add rice, and cook for 5 minutes, until tender. Attach herbs, and add salt and pepper to season.

Servings: 2

Bacon Ranch Brussels

Ingredients

- 1 lb. brussels sprouts, trimmed and halved
- 1 tbsp. olive oil
- 3 cloves garlic, minced
- 1 tsp. dried oregano
- 1/2 tsp. paprika

- ❖ Freshly ground black pepper
- ❖ 8 slices bacon, chopped
- ❖ Ranch dressing, for drizzling
- ❖ Kosher salt
- ❖ Freshly grated parmesan, for sprinkling

Instructions

- Oven preheats to 425°F. Mix Brussels sprout with olive oil, garlic, oregano and paprika on a large baking sheet and then add salt and pepper. Spread out your bacon over the pan.
- Bake for 30 minutes, until brussels is tender and charred.
- Drizzle and sprinkle with parmesan and ranch dressing. Serve hot.

Servings: 4

Best-Ever Gluten-Free Pasta

What does the xanthan gum do?

Xanthan gum and many other gluten-free recipes play a key role in this. It is made by combining fermented sugars and used in many foods as a stabilizer. It subsidizes gluten in this situation, making your pasta dough soft and elastic rather than dry and crumbly. It is a must-have and most grocery stores sell it!

Can I taste the dough?

Definitely! This dough will be fantastic with a few black pepper cranks, finely chopped herbs or a 1/2 teaspoons of dried spices.

Do I need a pasta maker?

Start by rolling out your dough as thinly as possible before cutting it (like 1/16 of an inch thin!). You should always eyeball cut the strips for fettuccine-style noodles, or keep the lasagna slices thick! Some other shapes are likely to be too bulky but worth a shot.

How long does the pasta last?

If it is new, you would instantly want to boil and eat it! If waiting for a couple of hours, cover with plastic wrap and refrigerate. And you'd consider drying the pasta longer than that. To do this, leave the pasta uncovered in the warmest part of your kitchen, on a baking sheet. The pasta will turn from fresh to dry overnight! Please keep it in a sealed jar for up to 2 weeks and enjoy pasta every time you encounter the craving.

Ingredients

- ❖ 2 1/3 c. gluten-free flour
- ❖ 2 tsp. xanthan gum
- ❖ 1 tsp. kosher salt
- ❖ 5 large eggs

Instructions

- Whisk the gluten-free rice, xanthan gum, and salt together in a large cup. Put the mixture on the pastry board (or worktop) forming a mountain. With your fingers, make a cavity similar to a crater. Add the eggs in the center of the flour.
- Lightly beat the eggs with a fork just enough to mix yolks with egg whites; then begin to incorporate a little flour taken from the edges of the crater.
- Continue to add the flour to the eggs, taking it from the walls of the mountain, then begin to soak the ingredients with your fingertips, until the dough is a bit grainy. Continue to work the ingredients with your fingers until you have collected all the flour and incorporated it into the eggs.

- When the dough begins to take on consistency, knead it with both hands: pull it back and forth with the lower part of the palm for a few minutes. Remove it from the worktop, scrape the dough residues that have remained stuck on the work surface and start kneading again on the well-floured tray.
- After kneading vigorously for at least 10 minutes, form a ball, wrap it in cling film and let the dough rest for at least 30 minutes.
- Take a part of the dough and form a regular ball, flatten it with your hands to give it the disc shape. Then roll out the dough on the always well-floured pastry board with the help of a rolling pin.
- Set the pasta maker to the widest setting and pass the rolled-out dough 2 times. Fold the dough in 2-3 layers and thin it again by passing it once more through the rollers. Repeat the operation until the dough is homogeneous and takes on a regular shape. Then squeeze the rollers and continue to pass the dough until you get a sheet of the desired thickness. The dough should be slightly translucent.

- Place the dough on a lightly floured surface and sprinkle with more flour. Repeat the process with the remaining quarters of dough.
- Adjust pasta maker to the desired with of noodles and feed dough through machine. Divide noodles into equally sized portions and curl into nests. Place on a parchment-lined baking sheet and cover with a clean kitchen towel until ready to cook.
- To cook: bring a large pot of salter water to a boil and add pasta. Boil, stirring gently with a wooden spoon, until tender, for just 3 minutes.
- Drain and serve with your favorite pasta sauce.

Servings: 2

Carrot Fries

Ingredients

- 1 lb. carrots
- 2 tbsp. olive oil
- 1/2 tsp. cumin
- 1/2 tsp. paprika
- Kosher salt

- ❖ Freshly ground black pepper
- ❖ 1/3 c. mayo
- ❖ 2 tsp. canned chipotle
- ❖ Juice of 1/2 lime

Instructions

- Heat oven to 430°F. Peel the carrots and cut them into 4 pieces lengthwise. Add olive oil, cumin, and paprika to the carrots.
- Put on a baking sheet in an even layer, add salt and pepper, and bake for 20 minutes, or until the ends are soft and crisp. Whisk the mayo, chipotle and lime juice together in a small cup.
- Serve sauce with carrot fries

Servings: 1

Cauliflower Mac and Cheese Drain Your Cauli

It might seem irritating after you blanch your cauliflower but to make sure it gets dried out, don't skip this step. The cauliflower liquid will finish thinning out your cream sauce, which you certainly won't want. Pat the chili dry with a towel or paper towels for clean dishes.

Use Whatever Cheese Combination You Want

We love how sharp cheddar and mild mozzarella balance each other out, but you can swap entirely in stinky Gruyere or creamy goat.

Do Not Skip the Mustard Powder

It may seem like an irritating ingredient to use in mac, but it's classic and adds a flavor depth you're going to want.

Ingredients

- 2 medium heads cauliflower, cut into florets
- 1/2 c. unsalted butter
- 1/2 c. flour
- 3 c. whole milk
- 1 tsp. hot sauce, such as Cholula
- 1 tsp. kosher salt
- 1 tsp. mustard powder
- Freshly ground black pepper
- 3 c. shredded cheddar
- 2 c. mozzarella
- Finely chopped chives, for garnish

Instructions

- Blanch the cauliflower in a big pot of boiling water until tender, 5 to 7 minutes.
- Melt butter in a big saucepan. Sprinkle over the flour, and cook for 2 to 3 minutes until slightly golden. Add milk and whisk until mixed. Stir in the mustard powder, hot sauce, pepper and salt. Let it boil, about 5 minutes, before it begins to thicken.
- Switch off the heat and whisk in the cheeses until completely melted. Move the cauliflower and whisk in cheese sauce until thoroughly covered.
- Add salt and pepper to season and garnish with chives. Serve.

Servings: 2

Broccoli Cheesy Bread

Ingredients

- 1 large egg
- 1 1/2 c. shredded mozzarella
- 1/4 c. freshly grated parmesan
- Freshly ground black pepper

- ❖ Warmed marinara, for serving
- ❖ 2 cloves garlic, minced
- ❖ 1/2 tsp. dried oregano
- ❖ Kosher salt
- ❖ 3 c. riced broccoli
- ❖ Pinch crushed red pepper flakes (optional)
- ❖ 2 tsp. freshly chopped parsley

Instructions

- Preheat the oven to 425° Fahrenheit and line a broad baking tray with paper baking. Microwave riced broccoli up to steam for 1 minute. Use a kitchen towel to ring out excess moisture from the broccoli.
- Move the broccoli to a large bowl and add eggs, 1/2 cup of mozzarella, parmesan and garlic. Add oregano, salt and pepper to season. Distribute the dough on the baking tray and form it into a thin, circular crust.
- Bake for 20 minutes, until golden and dried out. Top with remaining 1/2 cup mozzarella and bake for about 5 minutes, until the cheese is melted and crispy.

- Using parsley and pepper flakes to garnish, warmly serve with marinara.

Servings: 2

Cauliflower Garlic Bread

Ingredients

- ❖ 6 tbsp. melted butter
- ❖ 6 large eggs, separated
- ❖ 1 1/4 c. almond flour
- ❖ 3 c. riced cauliflower
- ❖ 1 tsp. Kosher salt
- ❖ 1 tbsp. baking powder
- ❖ 1 tbsp. freshly chopped thyme
- ❖ 1 tbsp. freshly chopped parsley
- ❖ 5 cloves garlic, minced
- ❖ Freshly grated parmesan, for serving

Instructions

- Preheat oven to 350°F. Section 9"-x-5" parchment paper loaf pan.

- Microwave cauliflower in a medium bowl for 3 to 4 minutes or until soft and tender. Let cool. Move cauliflower to a clean kitchen towel when cool enough to handle and force out as much humidity as possible.
- Beat egg whites in a medium bowl until stiff peaks develop.
- Whisk the almond flour, baking powder, salt, egg yolks, melted butter, garlic and about a quarter of whipped egg whites together in a large bowl. Blend until well mixed, then stir in microwave cauliflower.
- Incorporate the remaining egg whites and blend until it is ready to be added (mixture should be fluffy). Add the thyme and much of the parsley (save some for topping).
- Bake for about 45-50 minutes until the top is golden.
- Before slicing, allow to cool completely. Sprinkle with parmesan and more parsley before serving.

Servings: 1

Loaded Stuffed Zucchini

Ingredients

- ❖ 3 zucchinis, halved
- ❖ 4 slices bacon, cooked and crumbled
- ❖ 2 c. shredded cheddar
- ❖ 2 tsp. chopped chives and 1/4 c. sour cream

Instructions

- Preheat oven to 425°F.
- Put both ends of the zucchini off and discard. Line up chopsticks on either side of the zucchini, then make 1/4" slices meticulously to make sure your knife reaches the chopsticks. Repeat with leftover zucchini.
- Place the zucchini on a rimmed baking sheet with parchment, and bake for 10 minutes until pliable.
- Sprinkle the zucchini with cheddar and bacon, then return to the oven for an additional 8 to 10 minutes until the cheese is melted and bubbled.
- Let it cool a little, then top with chives and sour cream and serve.

Servings: 2

Loaded Zucchini Skins

Ingredients

- ❖ 1/2 lb. Bacon
- ❖ 4 large zucchinis
- ❖ 2 tbsp. Extra-virgin olive oil
- ❖ 2 green onions, thinly sliced, for garnish
- ❖ 1/4 tsp. ground cumin
- ❖ 1/2 tsp. Chili powder
- ❖ Freshly ground black pepper
- ❖ 2 c. shredded Cheddar
- ❖ Kosher salt
- ❖ 1 c. sour cream, for garnish

Instructions

- Preheat oven to 400°Fahrenheit. Cook bacon until crispy, then move to a towel-lined sheet of paper to drain and chop into small bits.
- Slice the zucchinis lengthways in half. Scoop out seeds using a large metal spoon, split each half cross-sectional into two sections.

- Move the zucchini to a large baking sheet, apply olive oil and mix. Season with chili powder, cumin, pepper and salt.
- Bake for about 5 minutes, until lightly tender. Top the cheese and bacon onto each slice of zucchini.
- Bake again for about 10 minutes, until the cheese is bubbly and the zucchini is soft.
- Serve decorated with sour cream and green onions.

Servings: 6-8

Zucchini Cheesy Bread

Ingredients
- 2 large eggs
- 2 cloves garlic, minced
- 1/2 tsp. dried oregano
- 3 medium zucchinis or about 4 cups grated zucchini
- 3 c. shredded mozzarella, divided
- 1/2 c. freshly grated parmesan
- 1/4 c. cornstarch
- Kosher salt
- Freshly ground black pepper

- ❖ Pinch of crushed red pepper flakes
- ❖ 2 tsp. freshly chopped Parsley
- ❖ Marinara, for dipping

Instructions

- Preheat oven to 425°F, and line a parchment baking sheet. Grate zucchini on a box grater or in a food processor. Use cheesecloth or a plate towel to wring excess moisture from the zucchini.
- Move the zucchini to a large bowl and add eggs, garlic, oregano, 1 cup mozzarella, parmesan, cornstarch, salt, and pepper. Thoroughly mix until well-blended.
- Roll the "dough" on the baking sheet. Bake for 25 minutes, until golden and dried out.
- Sprinkle with the remaining 2 cups of mozzarella, crushed red pepper flakes, and parsley and bake for about 10 minutes, until cheese is melted.
- Cut with marinara, and serve.

Servings: 4

Chicken Fried Cauliflower Rice

Ingredients

- ❖ 1 large head cauliflower, cut into florets
- ❖ 2 tbsp. extra-virgin olive oil, divided
- ❖ 1 medium onion, diced
- ❖ 1 clove garlic, minced
- ❖ Fresh ginger, minced
- ❖ 6 oz. frozen peas and carrots
- ❖ 1 c. cooked, shredded chicken
- ❖ 1 tbsp. chili paste
- ❖ 2 large eggs
- ❖ 5 tsp. soy sauce, divided
- ❖ 1 tsp. sesame oil
- ❖ 2 bunches green onions, chopped

Instructions

- Put the cauliflower in a food processor bowl with a blade attachment. Process into tiny rice-like crumbles, then set aside.
- Heat 1 table cubit of oil in a large skillet over medium heat. Add onions, cook for 2 minutes, and then add garlic, ginger, peas and carrots and cook for another

5 minutes, stirring regularly. Add chicken and chili paste and cook for 2 minutes, when vegetables have softened. Add rice cauliflower and simmer for 2 minutes, stirring frequently.

- Place rice mixture to one side of the saucepan and crack eggs into the skillet's open field. Connect the eggs with 1 teaspoon of soy sauce and scramble. Stir eggs into rice mixture until they are cooked. Stir and add the remaining 4 teaspoons of soy sauce.
- Continue to cook until heated and fluffy, for 5 minutes. Remove from heat and sprinkle with sesame oil and green onions. Serve warm.

Servings: 2

Magic Gnocchi

Ingredients

- ❖ 2 c. baby spinach
- ❖ 3 egg yolks
- ❖ 2 c. shredded mozzarella
- ❖ Kosher salt
- ❖ Freshly ground black pepper

- ❖ Freshly grated parmesan, for garnish
- ❖ 8 slices bacon, chopped
- ❖ 1/2 tsp. Italian seasoning

Instructions

- Melt mozzarella for 1 minute in the microwave. Add egg yolks, one by one, until they are completely incorporated. Stir in Italian seasoning with salt and pepper. Divide the dough into 4 balls and cool down for about 10 minutes, until firm.
- Roll each ball out into long balls, then slice it into "gnocchi."
- Cook gnocchi for 2 minutes in a big pot of salted, boiling water. Drain, and put back on the pot.
- Cook bacon in a large skillet over medium heat, for 8 minutes, until crispy. Drain fat and add spinach and gnocchi. Cook for 2 minutes until golden, and then garnish with Parmesan and serve.

Servings: 2

Cheesy Scalloped Zucchini

Ingredients

- ❖ 2 tbsp. butter (plus more for buttering pan)
- ❖ 2 cloves garlic, minced
- ❖ 2 tbsp. all-purpose flour
- ❖ 1 1/2 c. whole milk
- ❖ 2 c. shredded Gruyere, divided
- ❖ 1/2 c. freshly grated parmesan
- ❖ Kosher salt
- ❖ Freshly ground black pepper
- ❖ Pinch nutmeg
- ❖ 4 medium zucchinis, sliced crosswise into 1/4" coins
- ❖ 2 tsp. freshly chopped thyme
- ❖ Freshly chopped parsley, for garnish

Instructions

- Preheat the oven to 375°F. Melt butter in a large skillet over medium heat. Add garlic, and cook for about 1 minute, until fragrant. Whisk in flour, and cook until begins to bubble, about 1 minute more. Add milk and whisk until the mixture has cooked

- down. Boil for around 1 minute until mildly thickened.
- Switch off the heat and add 1 cup of parmesan and Gruyere, and continue to stir until cheese has melted. Then season with salt, pepper and nutmeg.
- Attach a layer of courgettes to the buttered baking dish, covering the slices of zucchini. Season with salt and pepper, and pour over zucchini around one-third of the cream combination. Dusting some of the outstanding Gruyere on top and sprinkle with the thyme over the cheese.
- Create two more layers with remaining slices of zucchini, a mixture of milk, cheese and thyme, as in the previous step. Bake 23 to 25 minutes, until bubbly and golden.
- Decorate with chopped parsley and serve warm.

Servings: 2

Cauliflower Hash Browns

Ingredients

- ❖ Kosher salt
- ❖ 1 large egg
- ❖ 1 tbsp. extra-virgin olive oil
- ❖ 1/2 c. finely chopped onion
- ❖ 1 c. shredded cheddar
- ❖ 3 tbsp. cornstarch
- ❖ 1/2 medium head cauliflower
- ❖ Freshly ground black pepper

Instructions

- Grate the cauliflower with a grater. Put it on a bowl and add onion, egg, cheddar and cornstarch. Spice up with salt and pepper.
- Heat oil in a big skillet over medium to high heat. Add cauliflower spoonsful mixture and shape into a patty. Cook for 5 minutes until brown and crispy, then turn over and cook for another 5 minutes. Repeat with a mixture of the remaining cauliflower.

Servings: 4

Cheesy Cauli Breadstick

Ingredients

- 2 cloves garlic, minced
- 1 large head cauliflower
- 1/2 tsp. dried oregano
- 3 c. shredded mozzarella, divided
- 2 large eggs
- 1/2 c. grated parmesan
- Kosher salt
- Freshly ground black pepper
- Pinch of crushed red pepper flakes
- 2 tsp. freshly chopped parsley
- Marinara, for dipping

Instructions

- Preheat oven to 430°F, and line a parchment baking sheet. Grate cauliflower on a grater until finely ground
- Move the cauliflower to a large bowl and stir eggs, garlic, oregano, 1 cup mozzarella, parmesan, salt, and pepper. Thoroughly mix until combined.

- On the baking sheet lined with parchment, shape cauliflower mixture in a rectangle, and pat. Bake for 25 minutes, until golden and dried out.
- Sprinkle with leftover mozzarella, crushed red pepper flakes, and parsley and bake for another 10 to 12 minutes until cheese is melted.
- Cut into breadsticks and serve with marinara sauce.

Servings: 4

Loaded Cauliflower Mashed Fauxtatoes

Ingredients

- 8 oz. bacon, cut into 1/2-inch pieces
- 1 large head cauliflower, cut into florets
- 2 garlic cloves, chopped
- 1 onion, chopped
- Freshly ground black pepper
- 1 c. cheddar
- 1/2 c. white wine
- 1/2 c. grated parmesan
- Kosher salt
- 1 c. low-sodium chicken stock

- ❖ 1/2 c. heavy cream
- ❖ 3 tbsp. unsalted butter, cut into pats and chilled
- ❖ 2 tbsp. sliced scallions

Instructions

- Cook the bacon in the oven for about 5 minutes. Move it to a lined sheet of paper towel; set aside. Drain bacon fat into the pan, leaving 2 to 3 tbsp. Discard surplus.
- Add the garlic, onion, salt (1 tsp), black pepper (1/2 tsp), and sauté for 2 minutes. Add cauliflower and prepare for about 5 minutes, until slightly softened. Stir in wine and stock; cook on low heat for 30 minutes.
- In the meantime, prepare a baking dish on a baking sheet lined with parchment paper and set the oven to grill.
- Move the cauliflower mixture in batches to a blender and add heavy cream and parmesan; mix until smooth. In the baking dish, add cauliflower mash and stir in the butter. Top with cheddar and broil for

about 5 minutes, until cheese is golden brown. Complete with scallions and bacon. Serve forthwith.

Servings: 4

Cheesy Cauliflower Bake

Ingredients

- ❖ 1/2 large heads cauliflower
- ❖ 10 tbsp. butter, plus more for buttering dish
- ❖ 1/2 c. heavy cream
- ❖ 3 cloves garlic, minced
- ❖ 2 c. grated white cheddar
- ❖ 1 c. freshly grated parmesan
- ❖ 1 tbsp. fresh thyme leaves
- ❖ Kosher salt
- ❖ Freshly ground black pepper

Instructions

- Preheat oven to 400°F. Cook cauliflower until tender, for 8 minutes, in a large pot of salted boiling water. Then drain.

- Butter a broad dish to bake. Pour half of the cauliflower and then half of the heavy cream over it. Sprinkle with half of the butter, with half of the garlic, cheddar, parmesan and thyme. Repeat the previous steps with remaining ingredients, and add salt and pepper to season.
- Bake for 30 minutes, until cheese is melty and intensely golden.
- Leave to cool for 5 minutes, then serve.

Servings: 4

Cauliflower Stuffing

This low-carb cauliflower stuffing shows you don't need bread to make a nice stuffing. However, if the party (your Thanksgiving Day feeding) is gluten-free or adopting a special low-carb diet, this is the only stuffing recipe you'll need. Plus, it's fully assembled on the stovetop, which bodes well for your oven space (more time for turkey and pie!).

Do not skimp on the butter

If you're going low-carb, you really can't go low-fat too from a flavoring perspective. When it comes to holding stuffing rich and tender, a generous amount of butter — four tablespoons is essential. Fat is awesome! Don't get rid of it. Use coconut oil or your favorite brand of vegan butter instead, whether you're vegan or dairy-free.

Create your land

Like any traditional stuffing, this recipe begins with sautéing your mirepoix — onion, celery, and carrot — which, when combined with herbs like rosemary and sage, makes it taste like Thanksgiving's. If the mirepoix is cooked, add cauliflower and mushrooms, which adds a little dimension to the platter. It is still fully vegetarian, but mushrooms and cauliflower bring a depth of flavor and texture to keep everyone interested.

Add tons of herbs

Cauliflower is essentially a sponge: it can soak up the flavor of everything that you cook it with, so we suggest going heavy on the herbs. Here, we have made a mixture of fresh parsley, rosemary, and sage. If you already have them on hand, you can use dried herbs (use half the amount of dried as needed for fresh in the recipe), but really, nothing beats the fresh taste, and a bunch of herbs usually cost no more than a few bucks.

Simmer

Pouring over some broth (low sodium vegetable or chicken) helps cook vegetables gently over the oven. When stuffed with a crispy shell, broil the casserole on the stove for 2-5 minutes after cooking.

Ingredients

- Kosher salt
- 1/2 c. low-sodium vegetable or chicken broth
- 1 onion, chopped
- 2 large carrots, peeled and chopped
- 2 celery stalks, chopped or thinly sliced
- 1/4 c. freshly chopped parsley
- 1 c. (8-oz.) package mushrooms, chopped
- Freshly ground black pepper
- 4 tbsp. butter
- 2 tbsp. freshly chopped rosemary
- 1 small head cauliflower, chopped
- 1 tbsp. freshly chopped wise (or 1 tsp. ground sage)

Instructions

- Melt butter in a large skillet above medium heat. Add onion, carrot and celery, and sauté for 7 to 8 minutes, until tender.
- Put the mushrooms and cauliflower, stir and season with salt and pepper. Cook for 10 minutes, until tender.
- Stir and add parsley, rosemary, and sage until combined. Pour over the broth and cook for 10 minutes, until fully tender and liquid is absorbed.
- Serve warm.

Servings: 1

Loaded Cauliflower Bake

Ingredients

- 2 tbsp. butter
- 2 oz. cream cheese, softened
- 2 small heads cauliflower, cut into florets
- Freshly ground black pepper
- 3 tbsp. all-purpose flour
- 2 c. whole milk

- ❖ 1 1/2 c. shredded cheddar, divided
- ❖ Kosher salt
- ❖ 3 cloves garlic, minced
- ❖ 6 slices bacon, cooked and crumbled
- ❖ 1/4 c. sliced green onions

Instructions

- Preheat oven to 350°F. Blanch cauliflower in a big pot of salted boiling water for 3 minutes. Drain, and squeeze water cauliflower.
- Make the cheese sauce: Melt butter in a large skillet. Add garlic and cook for 1mins until it is fragrant, then add flour and stir until golden for 2 minutes. Pour milk and low the heat, then add cream cheese and whisk until mixed. Take off the heat and stir in 1 cup of cheddar until melted, then add salt and pepper to season.
- Put drained cauliflower into a casserole dish. Pour the cheese sauce over it and stir until mixed. Add all other ingredients except 1 tablespoon of cooked bacon and green onions and mix together until well blended. Then top with remaining Cheddar, bacon and green onions.

- Bake for 30 minutes, until cauliflower is tender and cheese is melty.

Servings: 4-6

CHAPTER SEVEN

How To Speed Up Metabolism

Common Myths about the Endomorph Diet

Myth 1: Eat just fruit in the morning

Fresh fruit is undoubtedly a good choice and a great snack to eat. However, some fruits (including pineapple, watermelon, and bananas) contain a ton of natural sugar, spike blood sugar levels, giving them a high glycemic index. To prevent a rapid spike and crash, combine fruit with a protein or fat source, which will take longer to digest and help supply you with lasting energy. And while fruits are relatively safe, how much you consume must be controlled. Most fruits are a decent source of carbs. But if you are counting carbohydrates or trying to adhere to a low-carb diet, cutting back is worthwhile.

Myth 2: You speed up your metabolism by snacking

Your metabolic rate depends on what you consume, and not how much you feed. For example, in the context of "boosting your metabolism," you're better off not snacking than snacking on something unhealthy. Rather than concentrating on your eating frequency, concentrate on consuming as many nutrient-rich whole foods as possible.

Myth 3: Fat melts in coconut oil

Coconut oil has a standing for being the solution to all your problems. People use it as a makeup remover, as a moisturizer, and as a replacement for other oils when cooking and baking. However, simply eating coconut oil will not magically "destroy fat," as some myths believe. Moreover, eating too much (or eating it in addition to all your other meals for the day) will prevent weight loss or even cause weight gain, as it has 121 calories and 11 grams of saturated fat (which you should eat in moderation) per cubic cubicle (but could coconut oil be bad for your heart?).

Myth 4: Eating carbohydrates in the evening results in weight gain

Carbs are a source of food for your body, and your body can metabolize and digest carbohydrates effectively at any time of the day. It is always the total daily calories that make the difference. Carbohydrates, like any other macronutrient, can make you fat in the evening as well as during the day if you have a caloric intake higher than your needs.

Myth 5: Juicing's fantastic for losing weight

While juicing is an easy way to increase your veggie and fruit intake, it can potentially leave you deficient in calories, protein, fiber and fat. That's because, unlike smoothies, you get the juice from the fruits and veggies you're juicing — not the fibrous parts of the drink that help make you feel full to slow digestion. Juicing isn't inherently bad, especially if it provides you with nutrients from fresh produce; you wouldn't eat otherwise — but it isn't your only consumption of fruits and veggies.

Nutrition Myths

Myth 1: Cutting excessive calories helps you lose weight

Reality: Some people cannot eat enough or eat the wrong kinds of calories.

Many people are using food trackers and weight loss programs to predict how many calories they should eat per day. The energy balance equation states that you need to gain more calories than you eat to lose weight. Many overweight or obese individuals tolerate this lifestyle but don't lose any weight. What's the problem, then?

First, from a physics and metabolic point of view, there is a disparity in calories' perspective. Physics claims that a calorie is a calorie, whether it originates from a milkshake or an apple. Metabolically speaking, however, the calorie content does matter. Thus, apple calories are a better option for the general population.

Many who eat weight loss foods that are refined and packaged end up eating high-sugar and non-healthy fat calories that are not metabolically satiating. Even if a person eats less, with low-calorie, sugar shakes and bars, the body cannot lose weight. Most people "save" their calories for a treat or alcohol instead of supplying the body with what it needs — all the foods.

Second, the excessive counting of calories lacks the normal demand for food from the body. If people don't eat when they are starving or do not eat for long periods of post-exercise, their metabolic rate (RMR) decreases. As this occurs, protein (amino acids) is turned into energy instead of being used to rebuild the muscle.

Myth 2: **Food with reduced fat is healthier**

Reality: The most fat-reduced, refined foods add more sugar to improve the taste.

Foods with reduced-fat were once marketed as healthier alternatives than whole-fat foods. Because of this, several people ate low-fat dressings, processed foods and candy, thinking these foods were healthy and helping to lose weight. Food producers are increasing the sugar content to make low-fat foods palatable. It is also popular for gluten-free foods because eating starch flour without the extra sweetness is less than ideal.

Most physicians and specialists now recognize the need to consume fat, but it needs to come from the right sources — nuts, lean meats, balanced oils and avocados.

Myth 3: Carbohydrates make you gain weight

Reality: The excess will cause weight gain in any macronutrient.

Carbohydrates are the primary energy source used during exercise, from an exercise science perspective. Carbs maintain blood glucose levels and muscle glycogen levels, especially during extended workouts. Most people lack balance when it comes to carbohydrates or prefer the unhealthy choices that are fried, canned, or sugar-dominated. It is suitable for eating whole grains, fruits, and vegetables closest to their natural shape.

Any carbohydrate or protein that is eaten beyond what the body requires, or that can be processed as glycogen is converted into adipose tissue (fat). The average person should eat from carbohydrate sources 45 to 65% of their daily diet. Athletes that need more carbohydrate energy may be on the higher end of this scale.

Myth 4: Sweet potatoes are healthier than white potatoes

Reality: Both are dense in nutrients and essential to preparation.

The sweet potato has been promoted to superfood status in the last few years. As a result, people view white potatoes as "poor." According to the Cleveland Clinic, both sweet and white potatoes are nutrient-dense and provide plenty of vitamins and nutrients. However, sweet potatoes have higher availability of vitamin A. White potatoes produce more potassium, plus magnesium. Both potato varieties are almost similar in grain, calcium, and vitamins C and B6.

Food preparation is also essential. White potatoes are an excellent source of carbohydrates when boiled or healthily baked. We prefer to fry potatoes deep in the west or fill them with unhealthy toppings. Butter is not inherently a poor topping unless one eats too much. Typically, a little goes a long way.

Myth 5: Calcium comes only from dairy.

Reality: Calcium is found in many sources of plants and proteins.

Many older people are fearful of bone and joint-related conditions like arthritis and osteoporosis. There is no lack of dairy products inside the Regular American Diet. America also has one of the highest milk-consuming cultures and has many people suffering from the bone and joint-related disorders.

We are also told that products made from milk help develop strong bones. But there are plenty of calcium-rich, non-dairy foods that are healthy for our bones and waistlines. Foods high in calcium include rice, dark leafy greens, rhubarb, broccoli, almonds, turnips, Bok choy, dried figs, tofu, and bony fish. Increasing these foods while reducing high-fat dairy products can help with weight loss.

<u>Myth 6</u>: Vegans and vegetarians don't eat enough protein

Reality: The plant-based eaters consume enough protein with a healthy diet.

Some people think the best way to consume enough protein is by consuming meat and dairy. The debate about proteins is likely to remain a fight for some time, but this misconception arose because certain meats contain all the necessary amino acids (making them a full protein). And this contributed to the notion that eaters dependent on plants lack protein because many vegetable-friendly foods are incomplete proteins.

When it comes to nutrition, how much to eat every day and how much the body consumes in one meal is important to pay attention to. The average person can eat between 0.4 and 0.5 grams of protein per pound of body mass. Athletes need an increased protein intake—0.5 to 0.8 grams per pound of body weight. Equilibrating macronutrients and consuming protein-rich foods at every meal are essential.

Protein-related plant foods include ancient grains, nuts, peas, tofu, beans and some vegetables. Vegetarians and vegans can consume the necessary amino acids throughout the day or by combining incomplete protein foods; therefore, consuming protein from only one food source or in one meal is not important. One food can contain an amino acid; other nourishments do not. Beans and rice mixed, for instance, make a full protein meal. Remember, eating fresh, whole foods and well-balanced meals are essential to nutritional success.

Please allow me to clarify the above point before discussing how to speed up your metabolism. Metabolism may also be called our "internal fat-burning machine," and having a slow metabolism is likely to hamper our weight-loss attempts, while an elevated metabolic rate will do wonders for our waistline and our overall health.

It is being said that our biology will determine our metabolic rate to some extent, but there is a range of variables that we have control over. Simple improvements in our diet and activity levels will potentially provide a much-needed boost to our metabolism. So, there are no excuses; even though your family runs a sluggish metabolism, there are ways to increase it.

Exercising and eating healthy should be the primary priority. I can envisage you are rubbing your eyes right now and wondering if you're reading that right. That's right; I said more often, you need to eat. By eating, you stimulate your metabolism automatically. But you are training the part of your body to store fat by literally starving yourself (to be used for energy at a later time---note that your body thinks it is starving). And this can also lead to weight gain and, therefore, totally negate the primary aim of starving yourself.

It would help if you tried to eat food every 2-3 hours, probably 5-6 times a day. It will ensure that your metabolism runs as it should be, and this will also help you stop feeling hungry while you starve, which usually contributes to overeating. Of course, you will have to adopt a healthy, nutritious diet. It isn't just about stuffing your stomach with anything to try and improve your metabolism.

In addition to improving your eating habits, if you want to know how to speed up your metabolism, you may need to start working out. But the vast majority of people trying to either lose weight, burn fat, or improve their metabolism normally go the wrong way with this.

Indeed, most people assume that lifting weights can create a bulky body, so they spend their entire workout time on cardio alone. Certainly, aerobic exercise does play an enormous role in weight loss, but you have to work out with weights to improve your metabolism. Experts generally acknowledged and understood that resistance training is undeniably the best way to construct (and preserve) lean muscle, which will help speed up your metabolism.

You can achieve the greatest fat-loss results if you combine weight-training and cardiovascular exercise. Additionally, resistance training not only increases your metabolism but also helps you keep burning calories long after your workout is over. Many people who work out with weights will also lose calories for up to 24-48 hours.

It's also incredibly important to note that as you get older, your metabolism can slow down, while building lean muscle mass is a great way to improve your metabolism rate—another excuse to exercise with weights instead of relying solely on the cardio. You should also be mindful that a sluggish metabolic rate, such as heart disease, diabetes and osteoporosis, will place you at a higher risk of suffering from health conditions.

So, for those who want to know how to improve their metabolism, the response is easy— eating and exercising correctly and more frequently (especially with weights).

Learning how to speed up your metabolism is the first step toward your lean body. Nevertheless, making the recommended improvements to your diet and exercise patterns would certainly help you achieve your final objective.

Now, how exactly should you speed up your metabolism? There's a lot you can think by doing exactly that. Now you have no excuse to lie down on the sofa and do nothing at all. You can increase your metabolism and get an extremely healthy body in no time with these fast lifestyle enhancement tips.

1. Relax and unwind. You'd think you'd have to be super crazy to turn up your metabolic rate all the

time. But getting wound up or stressed out constantly won't benefit you at all. If anything, the metabolism will do just the exact opposite — considerably slow down.
2. Earn enough hours of sleep. Sleep deprivation isn't how to improve your metabolism. 7-8 hours of sleep a night can help the body burn carbohydrates more effectively and release hormones.
3. Don't throw away the day's most important meal. Skipping breakfast would only cause the body to conserve fat, thereby eating fewer calories. You can only improve metabolism by getting a fast bite before going out the door, and go about your day productively.
4. Always eats small meals. Frequent small meals ensure your body never runs low on energy.
5. Crash diets reflect a no-no. Overall, missing meals can only send the body into starvation mode.
6. Spice the food up. One way to grow up your metabolism is by a little kick in your food.
7. Snack on nuts. According to scientific studies, eating high in healthy nuts such as almonds can significantly ramp up your metabolism even while you're resting.
8. Job a chuckle up. Keeping your lifestyle generally healthy will certainly help you get your metabolic rate into high gear.
9. Incorporate a great deal of protein into your diet. It is very important, especially when you want to know how to improve your metabolism. Burning

protein requires not only more calories but also good for muscle growth.
10. Scaling up your workout. Pushing yourself past your normal morning run or scaling the work stairs will significantly increase your resting metabolic rate.
11. Fit into the workout routine with strength training. It is just as necessary to burn the fat as it is to create muscle. Together you can very efficiently improve metabolism.
12. Take supplements. Continue supplying your cells with the vitamins and minerals they need to work by consuming various nutritious fruits and veggies properly.
13. Drink lots of water. You can't emphasize this enough. Only how to accelerate your metabolism.
14. Place some ice over it. Adding ice to your water will increase your body's temperature, potentially helping you lose some of that excess fat.
15. Have a Joe's Cup. Black coffee not only gives you an extra boost in the mornings, but also produces improved metabolic activity in the short term.
16. Enjoy some green tea in the afternoon. Like black coffee, oolong or green tea contains capsaicin and caffeine for a few hours, which helps increase metabolism.
17. Milk is not exclusively for children. Studies show that drinking milk sometimes helps to burn stored body fat, especially in women.

Following all these ideas on muscle building and healthy nutritional eating strategies will help to improve your metabolism. Work your way through the list and better your lifestyle by using every single suggestion.

Speed Up your Metabolism and Eat More Often

What is even metabolism, and how does it serve its very function of existence? To learn how your metabolism can be increased, know the mechanism and how it affects your body, then read on.

Your body begins the process of consuming the food each time you feed. The nutrients are scooped up by your digestive system and then transformed into energy that sustains your body to function well. The whole absorption process takes 4 hours to take all the nutrients in a single meal. It will take your digestive system 12 hours to digest your 3 daily meals.

This reality means our bodies use calories in the digestion process. Carbohydrates and protein are more difficult to digest, so our digestive system consumes more energy. If your body's behaviors, like feeding, digesting, and consuming nutrients, have been accelerating metabolism, you can draw the conclusion that you have to keep eating to keep intensifying calorie-burning continuously. That may be another surprising truth you need to remember. But that is true. However, before you indulge in food that you have long set aside in your refrigerator, read on.

Skipping meals will cut down on how easily the body is consuming calories. So, eating more often helps if you want to speed up your metabolism. Indeed, consuming small amounts of food more often during the day will keep your metabolism going, keeping your body in a continuous state of calorie burning. Some foods, as pointed out, absorb more energy when being digested. These foods are changing your body's metabolic function. A few of these metabolism-accelerating ingredients include coffee, tea, chocolate, and a chemical found in chilies. But the speeding up isn't dramatic because the impact these foods have on how to improve your metabolism is just marginal.

Metabolism

Metabolism (or metabolism rate) is the amount of energy (calories) the body uses to hold itself going. Now a lot of these body functions are not even optional (like keeping the brain running). Some people will naturally have a fast metabolism (burning more calories) due to biology, age and environmental factors, while others will have a slower metabolism. However, your metabolism is not constant, and depending on your actions and lifestyle, factors can speed up or slow down over time. If you want to lose weight and build muscle, it is necessary to understand how to control your metabolism. If you want to lose fat and add muscle, you'll want to improve your metabolism to consume more calories, and you'll certainly want to avoid the number one error people make when trying to lose weight. It also slows down their metabolism and makes fat loss and muscle growth more difficult.

First Error That Slows Down your Metabolism

When people want to lose weight and add muscle, the total calories they consume as part of a diet (often a fad diet) are also decreased. It's true that to lose weight, you'll need to eat fewer calories than you are burning. However, if your body's too large, the difference between what you eat and what you consume slows your metabolism. If you are starving in the forest, this is a perfect adaptation, but if you want to lose weight and add muscle, it's a big problem. If you reduce the calories you consume by missing meals, this will slow down your metabolism even further. If your body isn't sure when it will get its next load of energy (food), it will try to conserve stores of energy (i.e., store fat).

How to Improve your Metabolism Diet

So, if you want to sustain or even speed up your metabolism to lose fat and add muscle, it's crucial to get your diet right. The following are things to remember:

1. Don't starve yourself; that's going to help your body burn fewer calories.
2. Most often consume small meals (e.g., 5 small meals a day, not 2 or 3 large ones).

3. Make sure you eat enough protein (protein has a complex molecular structure that puts extra pressure on your digestive system to break it down into smaller pieces). You'll also need a decent amount of protein in your diet if you want muscle production.

The Weight, Calories and Macronutrients

You have to understand how your metabolism functions if you want to eat more calories while resting. Many people blame their excess weight for their sluggish metabolism, but there are some quick and safe ways you can restart your metabolism and transform your body into a fat-burning furnace. Let me show you exactly how to naturally and quickly speed up the metabolism.

Next, you must stay away from any diet plan involving a daily calorie intake of fewer than 1200 calories. It is the minimum requirement the body requires to sustain its baseline metabolism. Anything inferior to that will cause your body to go into hunger mode. Your body grips on to every calorie you take in starvation mode and slows down your metabolism, making weight loss much more difficult.

When it comes to exercise, opting for shorter bursts of intense workout is always better than lengthy, low-intensity sessions. Why? For what? Since intense workouts provide a metabolic boost to post-workout, this will help you lose fat even after your workout session is over.

It's also really important to add a bit of strength training to your workout routine. Many people make the mistake of only doing aerobic exercise and don't understand that they appear to be hitting a plateau at some point. If you add to your everyday routine a little strength training, you can develop more lean muscle mass. Lean muscle mass needs a lot of energy to maintain, so the leaner the muscle mass you have, the more calories you can consume when you rest.

Another means of keeping your metabolism alive is regular eating. Snacking will potentially help you lose weight by making smart choices. If you make the right choices and keep your body healthy, carbs will help keep your metabolism up without adding weight. Complex carbohydrates will help improve your metabolism and avoid your daytime hungry feeling.

That is the problem these days with the highest protein diets. While protein is necessary to maintain muscle mass and keep your metabolism in high gear, depriving your body of carbs can slow down your metabolism and make weight loss more difficult. If you want to eat carbs, go for carbs that come from plant sources rather than sugar foods with no nutritional value.

So, in a nutshell, here's how to speed up your metabolism: remember to eat enough calories to sustain your basal metabolism, stick to healthy carbs and add some strength training to your workout routine. Recall both adding calcium to your diet and consuming several smaller meals during the day. This way, you will keep your metabolism up, and you will lose weight more quickly.

How Low-Carbs are Active in Weight Loss

A fascinating fact about gaining and losing weight is perhaps the recognition that while portion size matters, a meal's macronutrient composition still plays more significant roles. As a result, there are fairly many diets for weight loss, which have made the manipulation of macronutrients their priority. One such idea of macronutrient exploitation is carbohydrates and their usage in low-carbohydrate diets have been vilified to various degrees over the years but were still widely misunderstood by the generality of weight loss seekers. But then why all the carbohydrate fuss? What functions do they show in the body, and how can they and these low-carbohydrate diets affect weight loss for experts to have been involved in so many divergent debates about it?

Carbohydrates come almost entirely from fruits, vegetables, and grains, except for milk, which is the only animal-based product with substantial carbohydrate content. Essentially, there are two categories of carbohydrates: simple carbohydrates (which are more quickly broken down by the body due to their smaller particle sizes and therefore provide the body with the quickest energy source) and complex carbohydrates (mostly starch and fiber).

The human body needs carbohydrate more than any other macronutrient because it is among the three's fastest burning energy (with fats and proteins being the other alternatives), and it is what the muscle cells and particularly the brain is built to run on almost exclusively.

While all foods containing carbohydrates are generally metabolized to produce glucose, the body does not immediately consume all the produced glucose that is released into the bloodstream, however. The liver and muscle cells transform about one-third and two-thirds into a storage medium known as glycogen, while any excess is retained as fat in adipose tissue.

While glucose is the primary energy source of the body, muscles use glucose only for short-term activity bouts, particularly for the brain. On the other hand, glycogen acts as an additional energy source for the body and is only released and transformed back into glucose via the glycolysis process if blood glucose levels become too low or during any potential "fight or flight" scenario.

However, specialized cells in the pancreas secrete insulin (a hormone responsible for promoting glucose accumulation as fat in fat cells) to normalize blood glucose levels when glucose is abundant in the bloodstream. Insulin over-secretion due to the insufficient amount of glucose in the bloodstream normally contributes to increased body weight. And this is where the influence of excess intake of carbohydrates truly rears its ugly head.

Low-carbohydrate diets like the Atkins Diet and the South Beach Diet are based on the idea that people are not overweight but over-eating carbohydrates. Consequently, these diets are of the view that carbohydrates (especially simple carbohydrates) are so rapidly metabolized and absorbed into the bloodstream that dietarians get hungry so quickly after meals and thus tend to over-eat. However, this view of low-carb diet proponents, especially the Atkins Diet, created a lot of dissatisfaction as many nutritionists and dietitians thought that diets should be low in fat and high in carbohydrates, along with plenty of grains, fruits and vegetables, and dietitians should restrict their consumption of meat and other dairy products. While the experts' opinion became the de facto diet in the 1980s, the obesity epidemic also began to intensify with the generality of western populations, especially the American population, beginning to put on extra weight.

Nevertheless, low-carb diets regained popularity when people found it hard to lose weight and hold it off using high- carbohydrate low-fat diets. This revival interest in using low-carb diets was partially due to many small-scale studies that began to indicate low-carbohydrate diets may potentially be more successful in helping people lose weight. Several of these studies have shown that low-carbohydrate diets do not have all the adverse consequences that opponents traditionally associated with them.

Achieving Rapid Weight Loss Through Calories Cycling

When it comes to designing food strategies that promote weight loss, misinformation is abundant. Most people who aim to lose weight or change their bodies by dieting end up struggling, not because they lack the drive, but because they obtain misleading information about how to do so. There are lots of fad diets that we have experienced in the past few years that compel people to make dramatic changes in their diet either by reducing excessive caloric intake or by dramatically cutting out some macronutrients. These diets not only affect your metabolism but also take a great deal of effort. However, there's one option that won't require you to work harder on your diet or make drastic changes. By implementing a relatively easy-to-execute basic procedure, you will significantly improve your metabolism and your body. This effective technique is called cycling by calories.

Calorie cycling promotes weight reduction by continuously changing your eating routine by reducing your calorie consumption in 2-3-day intervals. You end up startling your body into a rapid weight loss scheme in most of today's fad diets, and your body responds by slowing down your metabolism so it can store fat for later energy usage. However, calorie cycling does not allow your body to completely acclimatize to a specific routine, and your metabolism, in turn, stays up to speed. With daily exercise, this helps you to burn off more fat.

How does this technique work, then? Let us take a look at one example. If you're used to a 2000 calorie/day diet, your body gets used to eating that amount of calories every day. With calorie cycling, you can slash your daily consumption by 400 to 500 calories for a brief period, about two days or so. Luckily for us, it will take our bodies around 2 days to understand this adjustment, and in the meantime, they can continue to burn the 2000 calories a day they are used to receiving.

Therefore, if your body still consumes the 2000 calories, you can feed in 1600, while it needs to find the energy elsewhere. As long as your diet consists of certain essential nutritious foods in the form of lean proteins, fruits, and vegetables, your body's insufficient calories will be used in the form of stored body fat. The advantage is that you don't need to make major sacrifices or improvements to your current diet for this strategy to be successful.

To be successful, this form of technique must be performed correctly, so you have to practice some common sense. Ideally, during such short periods, the calories you take out of your diet should be calories from unhealthy foods, mainly starch, sugar, and other heavily processed foods. Moreover, your calorie restriction periods should not be long-lasting, about a day or two before you return to your usual intake. The important aspect of this method is that by continuing to eat your calories, you will keep increasing your metabolic system's productivity. In other words, the metabolism will continue to increase over periods until it reaches its full amount of fat- burning! The result of that "diet" is that you don't die! You are consuming nutritious foods in varied caloric cycles, so your metabolism isn't surprising (and damaging). When your metabolism is in high gear, you'll start to see the stubborn fat blowtorched with daily exercise aids.

How Macronutrients Vary in Weight Loss

Each day in our diets, we move around these vital nutrients, proteins, carbohydrates, and fats. Some of us do this mindlessly, while others count each kilocalorie derived from those macronutrients. Pay a little more attention to the ratio of these nutrients in the diet for those of us who are on a weight loss program, into body-building, or who want to follow a healthier lifestyle.

To be specific on what the macronutrients are, these are substances from 3 main sources:

- Carbohydrates (Carbs)
- Fat
- Protein

We consume these three compounds in large amounts to give us total moving capacity. In the diet, we need certain nutrients to create and rebuild tissues, control body processes, and power our bodies through metabolism.

Each of these nutrients supplies varying quantities of calories:

- Carbs - four kilocalories a gram
- Protein - four kilocalories a gram
- Fats by gram - 9 kilocalories

Let's say you looked at a standard peanut butter jar's nutrition label, which contains 8 grams of protein per serving, and you decided to measure how many calories 1 serving would contain. It will consist of:

- ❖ 8 grams of peanut butter x 4 calories a gram of protein
- ❖ 32 protein calories

Your body requires 1 gram of protein per pound of bodyweight according to health guidelines. If you weigh 120 pounds, this is the equivalent of 120 grams of protein required in your diet per day.

The example of peanut butter will have provided you with 8 grams of protein. You would need to get the remaining 112 grams of protein, either from more peanut butter or other protein from animal and plant sources to fulfill your full requirement.

What is the appropriate Macronutrient Distribution within the Body?

Who determines how much of each nutrient that should be taken into the body to encourage wellbeing and prevent deficiencies - such as kwashiorkor and anemia? Since 1941, the scientific community has made recommendations about what constitutes a healthy distribution of essential nutrients for the average person. The National Academy of Sciences annually gathers a wide group of experts to discuss the latest research.

Recommended Dietary Limits (RDAs) are the guidelines but are also called Dietary Reference Intakes (DRIs). The guidelines' main component is the number of calories that come from protein, carbohydrates, and fats. The way macronutrients are delivered in the diet will either position you on the road to health and fitness or, conversely, create a state of ill health and illness. For adults, the Appropriate Macronutrient Distribution Range (AMDR), as a percentage of calories, is:

- ❖ Protein: 10 to 35%
- ❖ Carbs: 45 to 65%
- ❖ Fats: 20 to 35%

This selection is probably the most effective in avoiding the disease's risks and deficiencies while supplying vital nutrients to improve health and keep weight.

Why are Carbohydrates, Protein, and Fats Important to Health in the Long Term?

These macronutrients, including vitamins, minerals, and water are all required in the diet to survive. These vital nutrients have extraordinary, often mysterious roles in our bodies that we risk disorders and death without sufficient proportions of our diet. Here are only a few of its main functions:

Carbohydrate:

- ❖ They provide the largest percentage of the diet needed under the DRI.
- ❖ They are the primary fueling source.
- ❖ They are found primarily in starchy foods, fruit, vegetables and yogurt, and are essential for bowel health and waste disposal.

The body quickly uses carbs for energy; all tissues and cells use them.

Proteins

Were you aware that protein, after water, is the second most abundant material in the body?

Protein is needed for:

- ❖ Construction and repair of tissues - present in poultry, fish, dairy, meat substitutes, legumes, grains and nuts and, to a lesser degree, vegetables and fruits; fruit contains protein of around 2 percent
- ❖ Enzyme and hormone production to control body functions.
- ❖ Supplying carbohydrates to where the carbs are not supplied.

Fat

Fats are necessary for survival. They're the most concentrated energy source of which we need them for:

- ❖ Preservation of the cell membranes
- ❖ Natural development and growth
- ❖ Vitamin consumption (such as A D E K, and carotenoids)
- ❖ Inflammatory reduction
- ❖ Essential to healthy skin
- ❖ Regulating hormones
- ❖ Reduces cholesterol

Fatty acids are essential (omega-3 and omega-6) — the best fats for our diets. They can be found in fish and fish oil, nuts, beans, legumes, and organic vegetable oils.

How do I Achieve Weight Loss by Counting Calories?

To lose weight, you must:

- ❖ Be consuming fewer calories than your physique requires
- ❖ Increase the calories expended during physical activity
- ❖ Or do them in combination

The best way to lose weight without depriving the body of vital nutrients is to minimize food calories three days a week in a way that still meets general nutritional needs, plus 30-60 minutes of exercise. The appropriate distribution of the macronutrients described above gives space for adaptation. For example, fats are recommended for weight loss between 20% - 35%, so modifications can be made closer to the lower end.

Start by measuring how many calories the diet needs to encourage weight loss. Then consume the total amount of carbs, protein, and fats needed from high-quality sources. Combine your favorite exercises (dancing, kickboxing, Pilates, karate, weightlifting, Zumba, jogging, etc.) and watch the pounds fall. By counting calories, your dietitian or fitness specialist will help you decide how many calories you need. There are also helpful online calculators from reputable sources that allow you to plug in the necessary statistics to give you an accurate number of calories.

For example, a person would need to reduce 500 kilocalories a day for 7 days to reach a weight loss of one pound a week. As a rule of thumb, 1 pound of body fat (0.5 kg) produces 3,500 kilocalories. Using this rule, for example, if you want to lose 20 pounds (9 kg), you can reach your weight loss goal in around 20 weeks or 5 months. If we control the macronutrients in our diet, the basic principles remain the same. An example would be to add more protein to our diet for fewer carbohydrates. We will have equal calories while remaining within our bodies' optimal carbohydrate requirement, meaning that we do not eat unnecessary quantities that transform into fat. Understanding the macronutrients while keeping within the prescribed range can encourage weight loss, develop muscles, and maintain a comfortable lifestyle.

Conclusion

The majority of people who work hard but who fail to lose body fat are endomorphs. An endomorph is someone who has a sluggish metabolism and who is genetically inclined to store fat easily. Endomorphs are typically wide framed with medium to large joints, but not always. Endomorphs also have varying degrees of sensitivity to carbohydrates and insulin resistance, so high carbohydrate diets are typically not successful for regulating body fat. Processed and unprocessed carbohydrates containing white sugar and white flour are particularly harmful to endomorphs and appear to convert to body fat more quickly. Low to moderate diets with high protein carbohydrates typically perform well for endomorphs.

Although some genetically gifted mesomorphs and ectomorphs can eat whatever they want and never gain any weight, endomorph has to eat clean and healthy almost all the time. That requires the creation of high nutritional discipline levels. Endomorphs are the forms that appear to accumulate body fat very easily if they consume too much or if they eat the wrong foods. Endomorphs also cannot "cheat" and get away with it. Their metabolism is incredibly unforgiving. One or two trickster meals a week are the limit. They are often set back by bad everyday eating habits or regular cheat days.

Endomorphs typically have a very hard time losing weight by dieting alone. Often even an almost ideal diet won't function by itself since endomorph requires the metabolism boost that exercise offers. More essential for the endomorphs is a systematic approach to training and diet regarding fat loss. Even though they have a very difficult metabolism to lose fat, this book contains several exercises and training to help them lose weight in at least one week. Following the diet will help you easily lose weight and build the ideal body you so crave.

Made in the USA
Coppell, TX
19 March 2023